Paramedics: From Street to Emergency Department

Case Book

Case Book Series

This book is part of a new series of case books written for nursing and other allied health profession students. The books are designed to help students link theory and practice and provide an engaging and focused way to learn.

Titles published in this series:

Paramedics: From Street to Emergency Department Case Book
Sarah Fellows and Bob Fellows

Midwifery: Emergencies, Critical Illness and Incidents Case Book
Maureen Raynor, Jayne Marshall and Karen Jackson

Mental Health Nursing Case Book
Edited by Nick Wrycraft

Learning Disability Case Book
Edited by Bob Hallawell

Nursing the Acutely Ill Adult Case Book
Karen Page and Aiden McKinney

Perioperative Practice Case Book
Paula Strong and Suzanne Hughes

Visit www.openup.co.uk/casebooks for information and sample chapters from other books in the series.

Paramedics: From Street to Emergency Department

Case Book

**Sarah Fellows and
Bob Fellows**

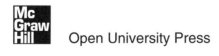
Open University Press

Open University Press
McGraw-Hill Education
McGraw-Hill House
Shoppenhangers Road
Maidenhead
Berkshire
England
SL6 2QL

email: enquiries@openup.co.uk
world wide web: www.openup.co.uk

and Two Penn Plaza, New York, NY 10121-2289, USA

First published 2012

A catalogue record of this book is available from the British Library

ISBN-13: 978-0-33 524267-2 (pb)
ISBN-10: 0-33-524267-7 (pb)
eISBN: 978-0-33-524268-9

Library of Congress Cataloging-in-Publication Data
CIP data applied for

Typesetting and e-book compilations by
RefineCatch Limited, Bungay, Suffolk
Printed and bound in the UK by Bell & Bain Ltd, Glasgow

Fictitious names of companies, products, people, characters and/or data that may be used herein (in case studies or in examples) are not intended to represent any real individual, company, product or event.

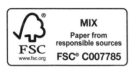

As it said in the opening paragraph "this book has been written for new and developing paramedics who want to test themselves". This is a great book written by a truly medical family, Bob Fellows with well over 30 years service as a paramedic and paramedic tutor Sarah Fellows a doctor and Simon Fellows just about to graduate as paramedic. This book will prove invaluable to the student paramedic and a great aid to the practising paramedic. It sets things out in a logical order, the case studies are thought provoking and give an opportunity for students to learn about situations they will encounter during their careers and experienced paramedics and practitioners the opportunity to reflect on similar cases and question their practice. It also gives an insight into what happens in the emergency department.

As a paramedic educationalist I would highly recommend this book.

Paul Bates (Paramedic), Higher Education Programme Manager, London Ambulance Service NHS Trust, UK

Individuals new to pre-hospital care will find this text well structured and clear. The informative introduction and subsequent case studies are written in an easy to read question and answer style. These provide a starting point for the reader to undertake further focused reading and investigation. A helpful text for students who are new to caring for patients, in the pre-hospital environment.

Amanda Blaber, Senior Lecturer, University of Brighton, UK

This book presents a series of medical vignettes of varying complexity. It discusses the differential diagnosis and clinical care, offering important background knowledge to assist the paramedic in following the best clinical pathway. Fellows and Fellows provide the vital link between the classroom and reality, removing the mysticism from the complex and ever changing world of pre-hospital care.

Dr David Zideman, Clinical Lead – Emergency Medical Care, London Organising Committee of the Olympic and Paralympic Games

Contents

List of tables and figures

Tables

Figures

INTRODUCTION
Assessment of scene and patient

This book has been written for new and developing paramedics who want to test themselves using some case studies based on typical pre-hospital presentations that will enhance the students understanding of the clinical method of learning. It also considers what might happen in the emergency department (ED) and so might be useful to new ED rotation medics who are interested to see the methods, rationale and thinking of paramedics bringing patients into the ED.

Arthur Fellows (1924–1992), my father, joined a large metropolitan ambulance service in 1950. The crews of that era had little or no training, with normally only a two-week civil defence training course and a first aid certificate gained within six months of enlisting. In those heady days, the crews had the three **P**s of ambulance aid: **P**ull up at the scene, **P**ut the casualty in the back and **P**ush off down to the local hospital. By 1980, when I (Bob Fellows) joined, it had been adapted to: **P**reserve life, **P**romote recovery and **P**revent the condition deteriorating. Today that remains true, with the additions of **P**aramedics **P**rioritizing the **P**atients with **P**rofessional **P**ractice, a methodology my son is currently learning as he commences his paramedic education at university, and my daughter (Sarah Fellows) will interact with a young doctor.

In this introduction we work through the different stages of a paramedic call out/shift and introduce you to some of the key things to think about at every stage. To assist the reader, an enhanced glossary has been included at the end of the book to assist understanding. Selected words are emboldened within the main text.

Priorities for crews before commencement of the shift

Crews must start by assessing themselves: Have they slept enough? Are they mentally prepared for the shift ahead? Are the crews fit and well and ready to handle a twelve-hour shift with potential for deprivation of food, drink and facilities? Will they be able to manually handle the patients following the use of a TILE (Task, Individual, Load and Environment) assessment (HSE 1992)? Have they set off for work in good time and allowed sufficient minutes to sign on, collect and check equipment and draw upon the drugs appropriate to their scope of practice?

The vehicle and equipment

It can be easy to make an assumption that the vehicle is ready, serviced, fuelled and with an up-to-date Ministry of Transport (MOT) certificate and a valid motor insurance policy. Other people in the health system background are doing everything to ensure that the chain of logistics is connected and provides a unified team response for the shift that day. The scenarios that we, as joint authors, have laid out in the following chapters don't mention repetitively every aspect that is taken for granted in pre- and out-of-hospital emergency care, in other words, gloves, footwear, goggles, aprons, disinfectant etc. As students and working paramedics, you become familiar with infection control protocol in order to protect both the patient and yourselves. Many large ambulance services have provided make-ready schemes where vehicles are checked, re-stocked, fuelled and washed every night in preparedness for the oncoming crews; however, some don't and so the ultimate responsibility lies with the **paramedic**.

The team

Crews can't guarantee they will work with their familiar crewmate or partner. Today they could be with an inexperienced relief who is nervous and looking to the 'senior paramedic' to lead the way. Maybe they are being assessed by a clinical team leader/tutor as part of regular ongoing **Continuous Professional Development (CPD)** appraisals. In all cases, crews are expected to act as professionals and they have to be prepared for any eventuality and be ready when the first call of the day arrives, usually when the kettle is first switched on.

The setting

Ambulance crews don't work 'out of the hospital' even though the public still think they do. Today they are more likely to start at a large ambulance station – often a hub for a district response team – with crews being dynamically deployed onto **standby** points for much of their shift. These locations are based on predictive software attempting to intelligently second guess where the next accident or emergency call might originate from, based on the time of year, the day in the week, and even the time of the day or night. While it's not always the most popular method with the crews, it attempts to assign resources in the right place at the right time to maximize speed and effectiveness of response.

The emergency call

The **999 calls** (112 equivalent in continental Europe) made in the following 25 case studies have been made by patients, relatives, other health and emergency workers and even total strangers. It's a crisis, and sometimes an emergency and callers require, almost demand, that the ambulance service races to the scene on blue lights in as few minutes as possible, whether it makes any difference to patient clinical outcomes or not. The reassurance of sirens and the flash of blue lights heading in the direction of the incident certainly has a psychological effect of calming the anxious bystanders, and, on rare occasions, makes a clinically significant difference.

The call is transferred from British Telecom (BT) (on request by the caller for an ambulance) to an **emergency operations centre (EOC)**. The call is answered by a dedicated, well-trained operator in the control room who has sophisticated equipment and software to ask the caller all the right things, extracting sufficient information to categorize the call for an appropriate response vehicle (DoH 2005). The clock starts ticking from receipt of the phone call and the ambulance or car must get to the patient's address in **8 minutes** if it's a high priority call. This eight-minute number originates from cardiac arrests that needed a defibrillator to the patient's side to stand any chance of getting a heart beating again in response to advanced life support (ALS). With ongoing changes to responses, crews have no longer than 19 minutes to reach a category B casualty in the same way.

On the way to the actual incident

Student paramedics are taught to state danger or safety when they enter a training scenario. In reality, what does that mean? They are trying to convey that they have, at least, considered safety as they walk into the hot zone of a patient scene. In reality, they are talking about dynamic risk assessment. Although not actually voiced at a real scene, all crews from beginner to experienced older hand are constantly checking and re-checking that it remains safe for them. If in doubt, get out and stay out until the cavalry arrive (generally the police, but it could be the fire service in a chemical incident).

En route to the call using either well-honed local street knowledge or a built-in satellite navigation, the driver of the response skilfully weaves a 3.5 tonne yellow and green (Battenberg markings) vehicle in between clogged roads. The medic responsible for driving the ambulance today has some exemptions from the Highway Code in relation to the 1988 Road Traffic Act, Road Traffic Regulations Act 1984, Traffic Signs Regulations & General Directions 2002, and the Road Safety Act 2006.

Progress and care is better than being cocky and casual. If we have a collision with a pedestrian or another road user, the responding service may need two further ambulances, one for the original call and one for this new incident. When driving an ambulance or a response car the key priority is for safety.

Crews get updates on a **Mobile Data Terminal (MDT)** that tells them any new information received in EOC since the crew were recently dispatched. Callers with very serious cases are requested to stay on the phone and the EOC will encourage the caller to put into place vital life-saving techniques in the meantime. This is known as 'hear and treat' and is a vital element in the modern ambulance world (DoH 2005).

Crews are mostly relaxed on the way to the call, partly because of the training but also because of familiarity with responding to what is to them 'their job'. Unusual or more serious calls naturally raise the crews' pulse as no one wants to be first on scene at a large 'multi-casualty scenario'. We have chosen not to discuss this type of major incident in these scenarios, rather, we have attempted to place familiar calls that require a mixture of knowledge and skills to determine the optimum outcome for the patient. A new crew would most likely see the vast majority of these 25 case scenarios 'on the road' in the first six months of clinical 'street' service.

In the final few seconds before arriving at the location, crews are scanning for clues. We describe this as the global overview and to some extent this continues until we are at the patient's side. What does the road look like, what sort of houses are there? Have crews attended any of these homes before or is this address listed in the register at EOC? All ambulance services keep a database of particular addresses that have in the past contained people who are violent or abusive to crews and EOC can pre-alert them to be cautious. The responding crews will be attempting to second-guess the ambulance equipment that might be required, the ease of access, the ease of egress (leaving the scene) and, inevitably, how they can minimize the blockage of a narrow street for the next 15 minutes by a bright yellow 3.5 tonne vehicle. It is not surprising that ambulances arriving on blue flashing lights attract the attention of neigh-bours and passers-by.

The ambulance service consistently dispatches a **rapid response vehicle (RRV)** to the scene, which usually arrives a minute or two before the ambulance crew pull up. Sometimes, on very serious calls, second ambulances are also dispatched, based on the caller information and the number of 999 calls received in the EOC. The scenarios you will read in this book are from the ambulance crew's perspective due to the nature of the book (i.e. 'from street to **emergency department**'). The role and function of the emergency paramedic practitioner has not been discussed in the book as the function of these roles is still evolving and indeed some services are no longer using them due to financial restrictions. It is accepted that there is serious pressure not to convey patients and to refer on to other health care personnel and this might be explored in a future publication.

It is helpful if the public can meet the crew in the street and wave them into the actual home or the block of flats as this can gain vital seconds. Callers are asked by EOC to move pets into a separate room; however, even with this pre-arrival advice (known as 'hear and treat'), the ambulance staff are often met by the family Labrador in the hallway and the television blaring out in the lounge. It is a regular occurrence for crews to be in a home while the family continues to watch TV as the elderly relative is on the sofa being attended by the crew for a new heart condition.

Arriving at the actual incident

When the crew have arrived at a street scene such as a **road traffic collision (RTC)**, they are very conscious of 'fend-off positioning' (which protects the scene from another motorist inad-vertently crashing into the rear of the scene) and still being able to get access to the kit in the side cupboards of the ambulance while being able to get to hospital if and when required to leave with the patient. Interestingly the police have started to re-label these incidents as road traffic incidents (RTI); however, this new term has not crossed over to pre-hospital care quite yet.

At the RTC, blue lights are left on to mark the scene and show other arriving emergency services the exact location. Crews tend to turn off the blue emergency flashing lights in the residential street outside the call, partly because they no longer need them in a side street, but also because they prefer to turn the engine off and take the keys with them. Ambulances have been stolen and driven away many times in the past by unscrupulous passers-by. Drivers of ambulances can legally leave the engine running at an emergency call, but this doesn't happen very often, even though modern vehicles are commonly fitted with a system called 'run-lock' allowing the vehicle engine to continue to run on its own supporting power and heat or even air conditioning and at the same time prevent petty theft of the ambulance. However, it doesn't feel quite so petty when the vehicle is removed from the scene while the crew are away from it attempting to save a persons life.

Selecting the appropriate equipment

It would be nearly impossible to highlight the correct list of equipment to take out of the vehicle on arrival and carry to the scene. The concept is that there is generally considered to be a minimum set which is most likely dictated by the employer to protect them against vicarious liability in the case of a defibrillator (for example) not being immediately available for a patient whose heart is in pulseless ventricular tachycardia or ventricular fibrillation. Broadly speaking, a primary response bag should contain a defibrillator, portable aspirator, dressings, stethoscope, sphygmomanometer, blood sugar analysis and temperature, plus an oxygen barrel bag with lightweight O_2 cylinder nasal and oro-pharyngeal airways, appropriate adult and paediatric oxygen masks and bag valve mask plus a reservoir bag for resuscitation attempts.

Paramedics also have a specialist bag with advanced airway management, cannulation and fluid therapy applications plus numerous paramedic drugs and the paraphernalia to administer them appropriately. Drugs such as **morphine** have special rules and only small amounts are carried and are often in a pouch on the paramedics' belt.

When the vehicle is outside the house it is relatively easy to go and get further equipment as required. When attending a more remote location with poor access, say a canal or cliff path, then pre-selecting all the equipment and carrying it to the patient's location is considered more prudent. This kit selection is enhanced with crew experience and is hard to actually teach. Most **newbie** crews take too much equipment from the vehicle and some old hands don't take enough.

Types of patients

Ambulance paramedics see two main types of patients: medical presentations and trauma scenarios. In both cases they still carry out a primary survey and then consider from that if they need to resuscitate. Following on from this will be a secondary survey and then a decision as to whether the patient is to be conveyed and where to. Initial assessment will cover the general impression of the patient, their responsiveness and level of consciousness as they approach, attempting to establish the chief complaint and obvious threats to their life.

Primary survey

The primary survey (for medical cases) generally considers the following:

- D   Danger
- R   Response
- A   Airway ⎤
- B   Breathing   ABC
- C   Circulation ⎦
- D   Disability (**A**lert and orientated, **V**erbal responses, **P**ain response, **U**nresponsive – AVPU)
- E   Exposure and the environment.

With trauma, we also consider catastrophic haemorrhage and any potential cervical spine injuries. Life-threatening problems are resolved in a strict ABC order.

Primary survey for trauma

Primary survey for trauma consists of the following:

- D   Danger
- R   Response and mechanism of injury (MOI)
- C   Control of catastrophic haemorrhage
- A   Airway with cervical spine
- B   Breathing
- C   Circulation
- D   Disability (AVPU)
- E   Exposure and the environment.

Trauma patients (special considerations)

By carefully assessing the scene on arrival it is usually possible to assess the rough speeds of the vehicles and thereby the potential injuries to any occupants. There are several triggers that will cause the first ambulance and medical teams to be alerted to serious trauma in an RTC:

- patient falling from a height of 20 ft or more;
- patients thrown clear of one of the vehicles;
- another patient injured within the car where there is another fatality;
- if the cutting and extrication of the vehicle might take longer than 20 minutes to release the patient;
- impact into the main compartment area of the car by 35 cm or more;
- any pedestrian or cyclist hit by a moving vehicle and thrown down to the ground.

Paramedics aim to spend as little time as possible at the scene of trauma; around ten minutes is the guide, if access and egress is easy. Early effective interventions, especially with children and trauma, are essential as it can be too late if the patient starts to deteriorate.

Physical examination is often conducted on the way to the hospital, especially so with major trauma as the aim is to minimize scene time and transport to a designated **major trauma centre (MTC)** and into the hands of skilled surgeons. A **pre-alert** to EOC to ensure the major trauma centre is available to receive further patients is a must in a busy trauma system after you have considered your trauma decision tree. Access to designated major trauma centres is not uniform across the UK at time of writing; however, roll-out is expected in 2012. In rural settings it is not unusual to have a 30 minute run on blue lights to definitive care. Several of the services experiencing these challenges enhance the paramedic education of selected crews to embrace extended critical care competencies. The initial MDT/radio report shall either be directly to the medics at the trauma centre or via EOC. This protocol will be directed by your employer; however, a simple tool is the acronym **ASHICE** (Fellows and Woolcock 2008):

A   Age
S   Sex
H   History
I   Injuries
C   Conditions
E   Estimated time of arrival.

'Hello ambulance service, so what seems to be the problem?'

Communication is the main element of human interaction. It involves both verbal and non-verbal dimensions. It also includes all the symbols and clues people use to convey and receive meaning. To achieve the best communication, all participants must take equal responsibility for their part in the process. Communication is only successful when both parties get the message. If paramedics are poor listeners they might make ill-informed judgements so I always remind them in training that they have two ears and only one mouth and should always use them in those proportions.

We benefit from seeing the situation from the viewpoint of the person experiencing it. Empathy is widely accepted as a clinical aspect of a helping profession. Sympathy, on the other hand, is the expression of one's feelings about another person's problem. Unlike sympathy, empathy uses sensitive and objective communication.

Patients must trust and believe that a paramedic wants to care for their needs. Paramedics can convey this trust to patients by accepting them as individuals. The paramedic should approach the conscious patient and make a personal introduction by name and title. 'Hello, my name is . . . . and I am a paramedic with (ambulance service). What is your name?'. Talking with the patient allows the paramedic to evaluate the person's level of consciousness and gives an overall impression of the patient's health state, though not necessarily a fully patent airway. It also may provide information on any hearing or speech impediments and language barriers. Eye contact is maintained in these early stages to ascertain responses from the patient that might not be verbalized.

Let us be quite clear, in the 10 to 15 minutes on scene, crews talk to patients and bystanders and gather vital signs. It is rare that crews have sufficient time to conduct a comprehensive health history, which inevitably will be dealt with at the emergency room once an assessment about the patient's priority has been made. Paramedics have to prioritize and recording a full medical history can easily get moved down the list in the emergency stages of pre-hospital care. Of course the crew will ask about the chief complaint and the present illness and even past history, followed by family history. They may even have time to discuss relevant parts of the personal and social history but this will not be in the same depth that would be required by the emergency department medics. A basic medical history is based around a primary, secondary and **SAMPLE** survey.

Elements of the SAMPLE survey

A sample survey consists of:

S   Signs and symptoms
A   Allergies
M   Medications
P   Past medical history
L   Last meal or oral intake
E   Events before the emergency (Campbell 2000; Dickinson et al. 2008).

During the scenarios, the authors have referred to the taking of a number of **vital signs**; for ease of reading they have not detailed in each case the why and wherefores of the assessment, but listed here are typical normative values for these findings, when recorded by ambulance paramedics. Paramedics are attempting to spot pertinent positives and negatives from both the history and the physical examination that help formulate a differential diagnosis.

Vital signs (these should be referenced against National Institute for Clinical Excellence (NICE) guidelines and various anatomy and physiology books noted in the references and further reading list) are:

- **Respirations**, (rate, rhythm, depth): ideally between 12 and 24, however, many fit and well patients consistently breath at 8–10 breaths per minute. The real issue is noting the changes, as we are always concerned if the respirations are rising or falling measure on measure. However, we will normally intervene if the breathing falls below 10 and rises above 30 breaths per minute.
- **Pulse oximeter/oxygen saturation**: ambulance paramedics no longer routinely administer oxygen to cardiac and stroke patients, but monitor oxygen saturation using pulse oximetry as soon as possible, ideally before hospital admission. The Royal College of Anaesthetists considers that supplemental oxygen can be considered for patients with an **oxygen** saturation (SpO_2) of less than 94 per cent who are not at risk of hypercapnic respiratory failure, aiming for an SpO_2 of 94–98 per cent. Clear update guidance was given in 2010 to all paramedics in relation to this.
- **End tidal CO_2**: the normal values of **$EtCO_2$** is around 5 per cent or 35–37 mmHg. The gradient between the blood CO_2 ($PaCO_2$) and exhaled CO_2 (end tidal CO_2 or $PetCO_2$) is usually 5–6 mmHg. In the case of $EtCO_2$, what matters is how it reflects the $PaCO_2$ value. Take, for example, a patient with massive head injury. You may want $EtCO_2$ monitoring and want to keep the $PaCO_2$ between 30 and 35. On arrival at hospital the arterial blood gases (ABG) are recorded as the $EtCO_2$ might not reflect the exact $PaCO_2$. They are best used as a guide as opposed to definitive numbers; for example, a sudden rise in numbers during **cardiopulmonary resuscitation (CPR)** is indicative of a return of spontaneous circulation, and the pulse can be double-checked to confirm.
- **Carbon monoxide**: a level of 100 parts per million (ppm) produces around 16 per cent HbCO (carboxyhaemoglobin) at balance, which normally is sufficient to show some of the classical signs that we expect to see (though some signs take some time to manifest, e.g. cherry-red skin). This by-product can be produced by the combustion of carbon compounds with an inadequate flow of oxygen. **Carbon monoxide** fights with oxygen to form HbCO instead of oxyhaemoglobin, which has a greater affinity for haemoglobin (over 20 times). High-flow oxygen will drive the numbers back down in time.
- **Skin**: looking for changes to 'normal' colour, temperature, and moisture. Skin temperature may be normal (warm), hot, or cold. Patient with febrile convulsions, and hypo/hyperthermic patients in emergencies can be checked in seconds. The dorsal surface of the hand is more sensitive than the palmar surface. Persons of dark skin generally have a high melanin concentration so there are differences in their response to light finger blanching or pressure during skin assessment. Paramedics should be able to recognize differences in patients with darkly pigmented skin and how this relates to their total skin assessment and evaluation. Abnormal signs may be **pallor** (decreased in colour), **cyanosis** (bluish in colour), **jaundice** (yellow–orange colour), redness and fever.

- **Pulse** (rate, rhythm, strength-quality): normal range obtained in carotid or radial pulses is between 60 and 100 beats per minute but it will be affected by a patient's age and physical condition. If only the patient's carotid pulse is **palpable**, the systolic **blood pressure** is thought to be between 60–70 mmHg. If both carotid and femoral pulses are palpable, the systolic blood pressure is between 70–80 mmHg and if the radial pulse is also palpable, the systolic blood pressure is above 80 mmHg. These are guides and it should be noted that there is little published evidence to support these indications.
- **Capillary refill**: the **capillary refill test**, although often used on adults, is at its most reliable in children under 12 years of age. It is used to assess inadequate circulation and possible impaired cardiovascular function. Pressure is applied for five seconds to the nail bed until it turns white, indicating that the blood has been forced from the tissue. While the patient holds their hand above their heart, the paramedic measures the time it takes for blood to return to the tissue. Normal return is two seconds or less.
- **Blood pressure**: this should be measured on patients when they are supine, sitting or standing, and on the right and left arms. Secondary readings should follow anatomical position of first reading if possible. The systolic blood pressure is the pressure against the arterial walls when the heart contracts. The diastolic blood pressure is the pressure against the arterial walls when the heart relaxes. Ideally systolic should be 120 or below and diastolic 80 or below. Subtracting the diastolic from the systolic produces a number, which is called the *pulse pressure*. Studies have shown that this number should be no more than 60 mmHg.
- **Pupils**: unequal pupils (**anisocoria**) might be a normal finding in some patients; however, generally pupils usually are equal and constrict when exposed to light. The acronym **PEARRL** indicates that pupils are equal, round and reactive to light. Evaluation of pupillary reaction is effectively an assessment of the third cranial nerve (oculomotor nerve), which controls constriction of the pupil. Compression of this nerve will result in fixed dilated pupils (Fairley 2005). The average size of pupils is 2–5 mm (Bersten et al. 2003). Abnormalities in size and shape of pupils could indicate cerebral damage; oval shape could indicate intracranial hypertension (Fairley 2005).
- **Temperature**: generally a tympanic value is used to record the temperature on the tympanic membrane. The paramedic pulls the pinna of the ear down and back in children less than three years of age or up and back in patients of three years of age or older. Normal body temperature is 37°C with a high temperature (pyrexic) being above 38°C in adults or above 37.5°C in children.
- **Blood sugars**: the normal blood glucose level in most people is between 4.4 to 6.1 mmol/L (82 to 110 mg/dL). Shortly after food the blood glucose level might rise temporarily up to 7.8 mmol/L (140 mg/dL) or a bit more in non-diabetics. Paramedics generally react to readings below 4 mmol/L.

Consent

Most of the time a paramedic discusses and obtains consent to treat the patient. Rarely today would any health care system ever do anything to a capable conscious patient that they didn't want, need or require. On occasions, the patient has to be treated when they are not able to consent to treatment, perhaps in an emergency, such as with decreased consciousness. Crews also are required to take on board the views of relatives as long as that is not to the detriment of the patient who is under the care of the crew who act as their advocates.

Medical direction

In the United Kingdom ambulance crews work to the requirements of their employer, often directed to observe national clinical **guidelines**. Although technically crews can choose to ignore guidelines and might sometimes have to, in reality, it is a brave paramedic who would work completely independently, avoiding both common sense of peer-reviewed published best practice and in the absence of real evidence, taking on board the consensus of expert opinion. Most crews have access via the radio or phone to further expert clinical guidance in the EOC.

On arrival at the emergency department

The ambulance entrance is normally separate from that used by the general public. Paramedics are expected to be bringing trauma and sudden serious illness that has occurred in the past 24 hours that is beyond the normal care of the local **general practitioner (GP)**. Sadly, crews often have to bring patients outside of those parameters and on occasion will take minor cases round to the **triage** area in the emergency department so that clinical need is prioritized in a very busy department. Crews can sometimes have to wait for long periods when the department is seriously backed up with cases, though naturally they will alert medical staff if their patient requires immediate attention. It has been the norm for many years that senior nursing staff meet and take a handover from the paramedics. Patients '**blued in**' to the department are generally taken to resuscitation (known as the **resus** room).

The handover

The crew, usually the **attendant**, give all the necessary pertinent advice to the nurse to ensure that the patient is taken to the correct area in the department and that the medical and nursing staff have a clear understanding of any immediate needs for the patient. Name and age of the patient are the normal starters so that the nurse can communicate comfortably with the patient and the paramedic. We try to ensure that the patient is fully part of this interaction unless it requires us to privately speak to the nurse for the benefit or safety of the staff.

There are so many different approaches to so-called standardization of information transfer by paramedics to nurses. There are dozens of acronyms used and each paramedic has their own preference. The authors are not attempting to sort this out in this brief text. One method used is **DEMIST** which is utilized in the following order. **D**emographics: name, age; **M**echanism of injury/illness; **I**njuries sustained/suspected; **S**igns as recorded (observations); **T**reatment administered, times involved.

Paperwork

The **clinical record** is recorded on what is known as a patient report form (PRF). This is often started when the patient is taken to the ambulance and information is transferred from their notebook on to the legal clinical record. Some crews write on their gloves with a biro; this is very old school and is unprofessional methodology, as you would never see a **Doctor** or a **Nurse** in the emergency department write on their gloves. The **PRF** is often completed at the emergency department after clinical handover of the patient. Crews are dissuaded by employers from spending long at the department booking patients into reception and actively encouraged to get moving on to the next case as soon as possible or at least in 15 minutes. The PRF is a multi-page form and one copy of the clinical record is left at the department so that the patient records are accurate and up to date with the actions and non-actions of the paramedics.

Clean-up

It is not possible to properly clean the ambulance at the emergency department. At best the surfaces are wiped over, blankets and bedding are changed and a mop used on the floor of the ambulance. Crews will often wash their hands in the emergency department in readiness for the next case, as ambulances do not have hot water or sinks.

Re-stock

Excess kit and consumables are carried on the ambulance sufficient for several cases. Practice varies with paramedics and their employers on re-stocking direct from the emergency department. Generally it is discouraged and on occasions an ambulance cupboard is in operation to re-stock from, but this is often problematic. In extreme situations crews will ask to return to station for cleaning and re-stocking, but often the pressure of work means this is not easy to facilitate due to the backlog of calls in the ambulance system.

Green Up

This is the term used by crews to indicate they are now available for the next case. Crews will usually push a button on their mobile data terminal to indicate they are now available. It is not uncommon for crews to drive to the hospital exit before **greening up** so that they don't have to use lights and sirens on hospital premises. The next case is the usual response from the system; if not, either return to station or go on to an active standby point.

End of shift

Although the crew will have a shift time when they are technically off duty, this is never guaranteed. Indeed a paramedic crew can receive a call with only minutes to go to end of shift, which will take them into forced overtime and the crew must respond. This can be frustrating to crews with a long journey home after a tiring 12-patient/12-hour night shift. Drive carefully.

REFERENCES

Bersten, A.D., Soni, N., Teik, E. (2003) *Oh's Intensive Care Manual* (5th Edn). London: Butterworth-Heinemann.

Campbell, J.C. (2000) *Basic Trauma Life Support for Paramedics and Other Advanced Providers*. Upper Saddle River, NJ: Brady/Prentice Hall Health.

Department of Health (DoH) (2005) *Taking Healthcare to the Patient: Transforming NHS Ambulance Services*. London: HMSO.

Dickinson, E., Limmer, D., O'Keefe, M.F., Grant, H.D. and Murray, B. (2008) *Emergency Care*. Englewood Cliffs, NJ: Prentice Hall.

Fairley, D. (2005) Using a coma scale to assess patient consciousness levels. *Nursing Times* 101(25): 38–47.

Fellows, B. and Woolcock, M. (2008) in Nancy Caroline (ed.) *Emergency Care in the Streets*. London: Jones and Bartlett.

Health and Safety Executive (HSE) (1992) *The Manual Handling Operations Regulations*, available at http://www.hse.gov.uk/lau/lacs/56-1.htm

CASE STUDY 1
Child collapsed in store

Case outline

A call is received to attend to a five-year-old girl called Carol who has collapsed in a supermarket and is now conscious but still very confused. The girl is lying on the floor in a crowded area with her very anxious mother seated beside her.

The mother mentions she had her first fit around 20 minutes ago and then a second one just a few minutes prior to the arrival of the crew. She is currently not having a **seizure** but is groggy and disorientated. On further questioning it is clear that the child has never had a fit prior to this and this has occurred completely out of the blue. She has been well with no recent illness.

As you begin to examine her, you notice her eyes suddenly deviate to the left, and a moment later she is once again having a **convulsion**. This continues unabated for nearly six minutes while you administer O_2, place a guedel (oropharyngeal) airway and support her limbs from hitting any sharp or hard objects.

Adult epilepsy affects 50 per 100,000 people in the UK. Convulsions affect 60 per cent of patients, with two-thirds experiencing **focal** and one-third generalized **tonic-clonic** convulsions. It is a relatively common call-out and children often present with chronic epilepsy; indeed sudden unexpected death in epilepsy (SUDEP) might occur with a frequency of up to 500 cases per year

---

1   **Status epilepticus is a dangerous emergency. When death occurs from this, it is usually due to which of the following?**

1   Head injuries;
2   Fractures of the long bones;
3   Dehydration and hypovolemia;
4   Stroke;
5   Hypoxaemia.

A   (5) Hypoxaemia. If this is left unattended it will kill, therefore there is a very high risk of this to Carol.

> **Hypoxia** refers to the level of oxygenation of the tissues. Hypoxaemia on the other hand refers to the level of oxygen in the arterial blood or a low oxygen saturation of the haemoglobin. The two don't have to occur together, for example, in a state of hypoxaemia you might not be hypoxic if your body is able to compensate for the changes.

2 **Given the risk of death to the patient, which of the following is the most important?**

1 Place a pillow under her head;
2 Apply restraints to stop Carol moving during the fit;
3 Set up an IV and run through a large volume of saline;
4 Give **diazepam**;
5 Open and maintain the airway and administer high-flow oxygen.

A (5) Opening the airway and ensuring that it remains open and then administration of high-flow oxygen therapy is a key priority. When that is resolved you can then move on to other interventions. Remember, ABC is the constant check on our care.

You administer 10 mg of diazepam (Valium) IV in an attempt to terminate her seizures. Approximately five minutes later, the patient's respiratory rate falls to 4 per minute.

3 **After several minutes in this condition the patient would probably develop which of the following?**

1 Metabolic acidosis;
2 Metabolic alkalosis;
3 Respiratory acidosis;
4 Respiratory alkalosis.

A If the patient went into respiratory depression you of course would deal with it immediately but if it were left unattended it would result in (3) respiratory acidosis, which of course would need to be resolved.

4 **What would you give the patient to treat this problem?**

1 50 ml of sodium bicarbonate IV;
2 Oxygen by nasal cannula;
3 Adrenaline 0.5 ml of a 1:1000 solution SQ;
4 Assisted ventilation with a bag valve mask or a demand valve;
5 There is no need for treatment.

A (4) Assist the ventilation with a bag valve mask or a demand valve to ensure that the acidosis is 'blown' off.

5 **What else would be advisable to measure while treating this patient?**

1 Blood glucose;
2 Temperature;
3 Oxygen saturation.

A All the additional measurements (1, 2 and 3) should be taken as they can all cause or contribute to the continuation of the seizure. Febrile seizures (2) are fairly common but unlikely to lead to a status epilepticus. Blood glucose (BG) (1) of <3 mmol/L can also cause the reduced consciousness. If BG level has dropped, give glucose, recheck and continue treatment pathway if corrected. Monitor oxygen saturation (3) for signs of respiratory depression, though it can be difficult to measure respiratory rate if the child has shallow breathing or has a reduced O_2 despite a normal respiratory rate.

Carol's fit is now controlled and she relaxes into loud snoring and curls up in a ball. You choose to continue her on oxygen as diazepam has a respiratory depressing effect and her semi-conscious level along with a SpO$_2$ of 94 per cent would indicate the benefit of oxygen. She remains in a **post-ictal** state until arriving at hospital. Children might experience a period of involuntary muscular contraction, followed by a post-ictal recovery period, often characterized by confusion, lethargy and, in some cases, profound sleep.

> **Post-ictal**
> This is a state generally seen post-seizure and is characterized by a generalized sleepiness with amnesia of the seizure events. The patient might also experience a temporary loss of function.

En route to the emergency department (ED) the patient is waking up gradually and after a few minutes she begins to talk.

6 **Which of the following would not be appropriate for the patient at this time?**

1 Administer oxygen;
2 Give fluid bolus to counter any dehydration;
3 Monitor the patients cardiac rhythm;
4 Administer more Valium at 5 mg IV;
5 Transport the patient to the hospital in the supine position.

A (4) Administration of more Valium would not be helpful as you risk a further respiratory depression and transferring to ED should be a main priority in case she returns to status epilepticus.

Further questions

7 **What is status epilepticus?**

A A seizure lasting 30 minutes or longer where the seizures occur in such rapid sequence that the patient remains unconscious between them. Convulsion, seizure, and fits are all acceptable terms used to define 'an abnormal and excessive depolarisation of a set of neurons in the brain' (JRCALC 2011).

8 **What other differentials must you consider alongside an epileptic seizure?**

A Non-epileptic episodes which can look like an epileptic seizure in terms of the movements caused and how they feel to the patient but are not caused by the abnormal electrical impulses in the brain. You cannot tell the difference by clinical examination; this can only be diagnosed by further investigation into the underlying cause of a seizure. Seizure-like movements can also be caused by acute muscle movement disorders such as acute **dystonia** or paroxysmal **dyskinesia**.

It doesn't matter what the diagnosis is in the long term; in the acute setting, you always treat the patient for status epilepticus if they are showing such symptoms.

9 **How do you know how much diazepam to give?**

A The dose for diazepam in children is 0.5 mg/kg (PR) or midazolam 0.5 mg/kg (buccal). This girl is five years old and, while you can estimate her weight or her parents may know, it is safe to assume you are going to require a more objective measurement. A simple rule of thumb is to use the following formula. This would make this five-year-old girl 22 kg and her diazepam dose 11 mg (PR).

Weight (kg) = 3(age) + 7 (APLS, 2005).

Alternative formula

Weight (kg) = 2 × (age) + 4 (Resus Council).

Key learning points
- Learn the key focal signs of a status epilepticus.
- Have a structure for how you would approach a status epilepticus.
- Airway management issues are a primary cause for concern.

REFERENCES

Advanced Life Support Group (2005) *Advanced Paediatric Life Support* (4th Edn). London: BMJ Publishing Group.

JRCALC (2011) *UK Ambulance Service Clinical Practice Guidelines*. London: ASA.

Resuscitation Council (2005) Edited by Bingham, R., Zideman, D. and Simpson, S. *Paediatric Basic Life Support Resuscitation Guidelines*. UK: Resuscitation Council.

CASE STUDY 2
Home is where the heart is

Case outline

Brian Price is a 67-year-old West Indian man whose partner called for an ambulance just after 3pm when he collapsed at home in his kitchen. On arrival, the ambulance crew is met by a neighbour who made the second 999 emergency call, as they grew more concerned about the condition of the patient. The crew go through a narrow hallway to a kitchen at the rear of the property on the ground floor. The scene assessment appears safe, with slightly difficult access/egress but it is clear that no trolley-bed will fit through the hallway. The initial assessment shows he is conscious but in great pain. The neighbour tells the attending paramedic that the patient has vomited. He is seated at the kitchen table rocking back and forth and appears to be sweating profusely.

The lead paramedic starts to question the patient who is fully clothed and heavy set, around 18 stone (115 kg) in weight. The patient tells the crew the pain commenced around 20 minutes before and that it has remained intense. It came on suddenly as he was standing making a cup of tea and is central 'behind my chest', the patient points at his own sternum. He has already loosened his shirt, which is dripping in sweat and his wife repeats that 'he looks like a ghost'.

The patient says he was admitted to the hospital seven months before, after he had had a heart attack and has since been diagnosed with congestive heart failure; his older brother also had a heart attack two years ago. He is belching and says he feels nauseous but hasn't been sick (contradicting the neighbour's statement).

Baseline observations following the medical primary survey are:

ABC:	fully alert;
Respiration rate:	20 bpm and regular;
Pulse:	120 bpm and irregular;
BP:	162/94 mmHg;
Temperature:	37.1°C;
Blood glucose:	normal at 5.8 mmol/L;
SpO$_2$:	reading is down to 93% so high-flow oxygen is administered at 15 L per minute by a non-rebreathing mask;
Glasgow Coma Scale:	15/15.

General appearance according to his wife, is paler than normal, sweaty and agitated. He has no known allergies and has taken one disprin tablet (300 mg) around 10 minutes ago, but hasn't used any glyceryl trinitrate (GTN) as the spray is empty and he hasn't got round to getting a new prescription. He takes aspirin daily, beta-blockers and a diuretic to control his high blood pressure and his previous heart failure.

Aspirin
It is recommended to give an immediate moderate dose of aspirin (162–325 mg) at onset of the heart attack as it produces an antiplatelet effect within 30 minutes (ACC/AHA guidelines). Contraindications are allergy or stomach ulcers.

One crew member starts to place the four limb leads and six chest leads in position while the colleague noting the BP sprays 400 mcg of GTN under his tongue, continuing to take base line observations and ask further questions.

The ECG shows 2 mm of ST elevation in leads V2, V3, and V4.

1 With clear elevation in V2, V3 and V4, what area of the heart is showing a possible infarction?

1 Inferior infarction;
2 Anterior infarction;
3 Lateral infarction.

A Anterior infarct STEMI

Inferior	II, III, and aVF
Anterior	V1, V2, V3, and V4
Lateral	I, and aVL V5, and V6

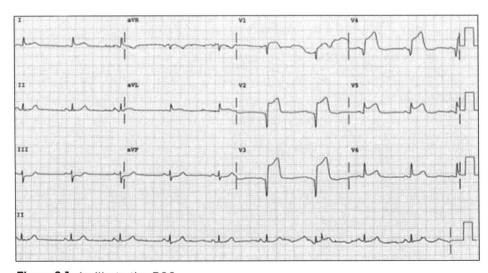

Figure 2.1 An illustrative ECG

2 **What is your current basic differential diagnosis?**

A The symptoms and ECG point towards an acute coronary syndrome (chest pain) rather than stable angina (pain on exertion). This is an umbrella term covering the following:

* unstable angina;
* non-ST elevation myocardial infarction;
* ST elevation myocardial infarction (STEMI).

Unstable angina: the patient is likely to have a history of worsening angina although this might be the first instance of spontaneous chest pain at rest. It is characterized by pain occurring at rest due to a small thrombus causing obstruction to vessels but not producing complete occlusion (myocardial infarction).

ST elevation MI and non-ST elevation MI: these will present with the same symptoms. Likely to have a history of angina and associated cardiac problems, although this is not definitive.

Other types of 'chest pain' to consider are:

* 'Radiating to the back': dissecting or enlarging thoracic aortic aneurysm.
* 'Worse on inspiration or movement': pleuritic chest pain associated with a pulmonary embolism, costochondritis or pericarditis (also relieved by sitting forward).

3 **What is the pathophysiology behind acute coronary syndrome?**

A Atherosclerotic lesions are covered by a fibrous cap which, when ruptured or eroded, can release pro-coagulant debris. This leads to platelet aggregation and downstream blockage of smaller arteries (in this case coronary arteries). Serotonin and thromboxane released from the platelets also causes vasoconstriction, overall reducing coronary blood flow.

4 **What are the risk factors that increase the chances of suffering from coronary heart disease?**

A Increasing age, high BP, obesity, family history of ischaemic heart disease, stress, diabetes, smoking, high cholesterol and male gender.

5 **Given the initial signs and symptoms, is it likely that Brian Price has suffered a second heart attack?**

A It is possible that given his past medical history Mr Price could be experiencing unstable angina but, with no chest pain since his previous heart attack and the sudden onset of the symptoms and ST elevation on three adjoining leads on his recent ECG, it is more likely that he is suffering from a myocardial infarction. The cardiac/emergency department will carry out further ECGs and take blood to assess his cardiac markers such as the levels of his troponins.

6 **What other signs and symptoms might you expect in an acute myocardial infarction?**

A Patients will often be extremely anxious and can sometimes describe an impending sense of doom. The panic created by these feelings alongside the pain tend to cause an increase in blood pressure, although you may also see a drop in blood pressure in some cases where the damage to the heart leads to a reduced cardiac output. You will generally note a tachycardia as the pain and stress drives up the heart rate but look out for bradycardia and also heart block caused by the infarct region.

While the patient here is experiencing the classic pain presentation, diabetic or elderly patients can experience a silent MI with symptoms like dyspnoea and nausea to point to the problem or it may lead to more severe symptoms associated with the drop in cardiac output (pulmonary oedema, hypotension and loss of consciousness). The pain presentation might not always be as straightforward, with some mistaking the pain for indigestion but with it not being relieved by antacids or body movement.

Women also experience variations in symptoms with nausea, epigastric discomfort and exhaustion. Because their symptoms are less clear cut, some women tend to ignore or under-estimate their symptoms.

Table 2.1 Shows a list of differences between angina and MI.

7 **What would be your management plan at this point?**

A Following administration of 400 mcgs of glyceryl trinitrate spray (GTN) under the patients tongue, an 18 gauge cannula is placed into the right arm and flushed through. The patient is then administered 5 mg of morphine which has been diluted with sodium chloride (0.9%), to ensure a concentration of 1 mg in 1 ml. The morphine is administered slowly to the patient while you carefully monitor them, with a standby injection of 400 mcgs of naloxone just in case of severe respiratory depression. His blood pressure is re-taken (150/88) and his oxygen reduced to a nasal cannula at 4 litres per minute as his oxygen saturation has risen to 95 per cent.

> Brian states his pain is reduced and is recorded as 7 on the pain scale compared to a 10 when the crew arrived on scene.

Table 2.1 Difference between angina and MI

Angina	MI
Mild to moderate pain in the retro-sternal region, radiates to arm, epigastrium, and neck	Pain will have the same pattern as angina but might be more severe
Precipitated by exercise or stress	Often occurs at rest as well as during exercise and stress
Relieved by rest/nitrates	No relief from pain
Mild anxiety	Severe anxiety
No signs of increased sympathetic activity	Increased sympathetic activity
No nausea or vomiting	Nausea and vomiting are common

8 **How does GTN reduce symptoms of chest pain?**

A Glyceryl trinitrate causes vasodilation and some smooth muscle relaxation to reduce the pre-load on the heart and so reduces the oxygen consumption of the myocardium. It also relieves coronary spasm and increases circulation to ischaemic regions to relieve the symptoms. It is more effective on partial occlusions (as in angina) and so in infarctions often provides very little relief.

Key learning points

- Recognize the key symptoms of a STEMI and be aware of any further ECG changes that occur en route to hospital.
- Make sure you print off copies to hand over with the patient (our illustrative ECG deliberately has no name on it). Yours will include D.O.B. and time of print.
- Gain an understanding of the different types of chest pain that can present and how your differential diagnosis might change with each.

REFERENCE

ACC/AHA (2004) *Guidelines for the Management of Patients With ST-Elevation Myocardial Infarction: Executive Summary.*

Case outline

Bob Thompson is a 48-year-old West Midlands man whose partner called for an ambulance just before 9 pm when he collapsed at home in his study.

On arrival, the ambulance crew is met by a middle-aged man who made the second 999 call as he grew more concerned about Bob. The ambulance crew enter the property and are shown into a study at the front of the house on the ground floor. The **global overview** shows a safe scene with a challenging access and narrow doorway close to a desk, allowing a chair at best to fit through the hallway into the study. Bob's partner, John, explains to the attendant paramedic that Bob has been unwell since the morning, feeling breathless and wheezy but had insisted he didn't need to go to hospital. When Bob became progressively worse and found it difficult to speak, John decided to call an ambulance against his partner's wishes.

On initial observation, Bob is conscious and sat in a leather chair leaning forward and appears to be quite pale and sweaty. Through pursed lips Bob attempts to speak but struggles to complete a simple sentence without pausing for breath. His breathing is fast and somewhat laboured as he tries to explain that he 'can't catch his breath'. Next to him lying on the desk is a blue inhaler that Bob has tried to take throughout the day but has done nothing to improve his symptoms.

Bob, who is medium set in build at around 15 stones, has an open neck shirt on and his muscles on his upper chest and neck are clearly straining as he attempts to exhale each of his shallow breaths.

John assists the crew by filling in some of the background history stating that Bob has not had a serious asthma attack for at least 18 months and that he believes Bob is under severe stress at work with deadlines and working late. He says he has been struggling though a mild cold but has not been sufficiently unwell to miss work.

> **Global overview**
> Active reflective model (in action) of the patient's situation and how it will affect the paramedic's method of approach and initial actions.

> **Tips**
> Assist the ventilation with some high-flow oxygen connected to a BVM if ventilation rate is <10 or >30 or if O_2 saturations are <90%. Expect COPD patients to run with low O_2 sats.

Baseline observations following the primary survey are:

Airway: clear and dry with no obstruction or wheeze
Respiration rate: 24 bpm (shallow using accessory muscles)
Pulse: 140 bpm
BP: 136/80 mmHg
Temperature: 37.0°C
Blood glucose: 5.6 mmol/L (last meal eight hours ago)
SpO$_2$:   94%
Peak Expiratory Flow (PEF): 50% of best available score

Breathing assessment (inspection, palpation, percussion, auscultation): conduct an assessment for colour of the skin and for any evidence of cyanosis, peripherally and centrally. Oxygen is administered to Bob at 15 L per minute, due to the low SpO$_2$ by a non-rebreathing mask.

Peak flow
Acute asthma is often seen as 33–50 per cent of the best predicted best value which gives you a rough guide in the absence of any known previous best readings. (Normal practice is to select the best of three readings if the patient is able; BTS guidelines 2008).

1   **Which inhaler colours correlate to the drug administered?**

A   Patients generally know the colour of their inhaler rather than what it contains so this will help you determine what they might be on (see Table 3.1). Also remember to gather inhalers along with medications to take to hospital as there are still variations on each colour. Also, inhalers can be broken, out of date or empty so by taking them to the hospital with you, a problem like this may help explain why a patient cannot get control of their symptoms.

Table 3.1 Guide to inhalers

Inhaler colour	Action	Drug
BLUE	Reliever – short-acting Beta-agonist	salbutamol (Ventolin)
		terbutaline (Bricanyl)
GREEN	Long-acting Beta-agonist	eformoterol (Oxis)
		salmeterol (Serevent)
PURPLE	Long-acting Beta-agonist/	Seretide (fluticasone/salmeterol)
RED	Corticosteroid combination	Symbicort (budesonide/eformoterol)
WHITE		
BROWN	Preventers – Corticosteroid	beclomethasone (Becotide)
ORANGE		budesonide (Pulmicort)
BURGUNDY		fluticasone (Flixotide)

The paramedic asks Bob if it is OK to open his shirt and therefore expose the chest to observe front wall movement. Bilateral chest wall movement is occurring but expansion is inadequate. At this point you need to be concerned about signs of fatigue in the patient as he has been struggling for breath for most of the day and there is a risk he might go into respiratory arrest.

There is some wheezing on expiration with no **stridor** heard by auscultation using a stethoscope (higher pitched noise on inspiration suggestive of upper respiratory obstruction). The position of the trachea is midline and its location in the suprasternal notch is normal.

The paramedic continues to listen to the chest with a stethoscope asking Bob to breathe in and out through his mouth while he listens on both sides of the chest, fourth intercostal space in the mid-clavicular line and in the mid-axilla under the arm-pit at the rear of the chest and below the shoulder blade.

The attendant is generally listening for:

* normal or reduced air entry;
* equal air entry on each side;
* wheezing (on inspiration and/or expiration).

There is no sound of **crepitations** at the rear of the chest. These would sound as **crackles,** heard low down in the lung fields at the rear and indicate fluid in the lung.

General appearance

Bob is paler than normal according to John, and is clearly very tired and moving slowly. Although he is allergic to peanuts he doesn't believe he has actually been in contact with them for months. He has been taking 500 mg of **paracetamol** every six hours for the past three days for his cold and his temperature has returned to normal today. He has however been taking his inhalers more frequently over the past few days and has been waking at night feeling breathless. He has never had any known heart problems or diabetes.

The ambulance technician re-checks Bob's SpO_2 reading (now 95%) and switches to a 2 L nasal cannula with built-in end tidal CO_2 attaching the BP cuff to his right arm and a set of four limb leads (NSR) and allows the attending paramedic to ask further questions. The aim at this point is to maintain Bob's SpO_2 at >95%.

2   **What is your current basic differential diagnosis?**

A
* Acute asthma crisis (most likely);
* Anaphylactic reaction (known peanut allergy, possibility of other unknown allergies);
* Pulmonary embolism (long-term coughing, pain in chest wall);
* Spontaneous pneumothorax (cough and cold, difficulty in breathing, pneumonia);
* Chest pain;
* Silent MI (VERY important to consider in elderly or diabetic).

3   **How do we differentiate between these options and why?**

A   A thorough history will help identify possible causes of dyspnoea. In particular, it is important to ask the patient about:

- **The length of time they have had difficulty breathing.**
  Asthma is often slowly progressive over about six hours but can also occur suddenly such as when exposed to an **allergen** or after exercise. Sudden onset is more suggestive of a PE, **pneumothorax** or **anaphylaxis**.
- **Is there any pain associated with the patients breathing?**
  Pain with breathlessness is mostly suggestive of a PE or an MI (except silent MI). Any pain can cause discomfort though and don't rule out a diagnosis based on the presence or absence of pain.
- **Does the patient have a cough/recent illness?**
  Recent illness is associated with an acute exacerbation of asthma; tension pneumothorax can also be secondary to pneumonia. A productive cough of green/yellow sputum suggests an infection (bronchitis, pneumonia, chest infection) whereas asthmatics tend to produce clear or whitish sputum as normal.

Table 3.2 Most common findings of the differential diagnosis (Ddx)

	History	*Signs & symptoms*
Pneumonia	Ischaemic heart disease (IHD), smoker	Dyspnoea, fever, cough and tachycardia
Pulmonary embolism	Immobilization, recent surgery thrombotic disease	Dyspnoea, pleuritic chest pain, cough, leg pain, leg **oedema**, tachycardia, tachypnoea, fever
LVF	IHD hypertension	**Dyspnoea**, especially on exertion, **orthopnoea**/nocturnal dyspnoea, peripheral oedema, raised jugular vein pressure (JVP), tachycardia, progressive symptoms
Asthma	Previous asthma, recent sharp increase in inhaler use and allergen exposure	Dyspnoea, cough, unable to complete sentences, wheezing, tachypnoea, tachycardia, pulsus paradoxus, hyperresonant chest, accessory muscle use, PEF<50% normal

4 **Based on the examination and current findings, what is your final diagnosis?**

A Acute asthma attack is the most likely.

5 **What is the pathophysiology behind asthma?**

A Asthma is caused by a chronic inflammation of the bronchi, making them narrower. The muscles around the bronchi become irritated and contract, causing sudden worsening of the symptoms. The inflammation can also cause the mucus glands to produce excessive sputum which further blocks the air passages, a very common presentation.

6 **What would be your management plan at this point?**

A Your management plan would be:

- Salbutamol 5 mg via nebulizer (6–8 L/min);

- If there is no improvement to the peak flow reading, repeat dose after 5 minutes;
- There is no limit to the number of repeats but stop if side effects occur (extreme tachycardia >140 beats per minute in adults, tremors etc.);
- In acute severe or life-threatening asthma add **ipratropium bromide** and IM **adrenaline** 1:000;
- Obtain IV access if possible;
- Peak flow recordings (pre- and post-drug administration) are very useful if patient can handle this.

7 **How does Ventolin/salbutamol reduce symptoms of asthma?**

A **Salbutamol** is a β2-adrenoceptor agonist and causes a relaxation of muscles leading to bronchodilation (widens bronchioles) to make expiration easier. It also inhibits mast cells from releasing inflammatory mediators thus reducing inflammation of the airway.

Key learning points

Asthma in its severest form can be life threatening and is often associated with comorbidities that increase the likelihood of a poor outcome. You must have a clear management strategy and have a range of treatment options in case the patient doesn't respond to normal medication protocols.

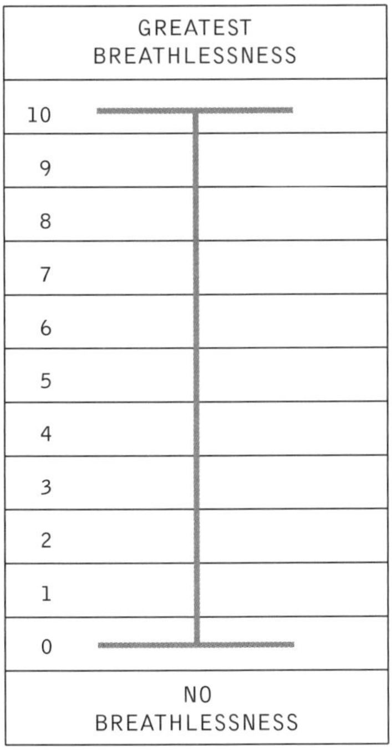

Visual Analogue Scale
Used by patients to show the carer how they feel, useful when speech is very difficult due to breathlessness (Frownfelter and Ryan 2000).

Figure 3.1 Breathlessness scale

REFERENCES

British Thoracic Society (BTS) (2008) *British Guideline on the Management of Asthma: A National Clinical Guideline.* London: BTS.

Frownfelter, D. and Ryan, J. (2000) Dyspnea: measurement and evaluation. *Cardiopulmonary Physical Therapy Journal* 11(1): 7–15.

Huffin' and puffin'

Case outline

It is not unusual to attend a regular caller, someone that is reasonably well known to the local crews who visit the patient's address on a frequent basis. Mrs Gladys Underhill had difficulty in breathing and her son, who was visiting his mother, called the ambulance from the house phone.

The ambulance arrived and pulled up outside the home where her son came out of the house to meet them. This is sometimes helpful if the patient is not time critical as it allows the crew to talk to the relative and get a global overview away from the ears of the patient. Her son mentions she seems to be more confused than normal and has been coughing more than usual, but he thinks it is to do with her breathlessness.

Gladys, who is 76 years of age, has been a smoker all her life and is now effectively housebound and on home oxygen for the difficult crises that are becoming more regular and have now exacerbated to almost daily. The crew have selected appropriate equipment for a primary response, including their own O_2 set and walked down to the rear of the terraced property. Gladys is sat at the kitchen table leaning forward with a nasal cannula on her face that was set to 24% on 2 L of oxygen flow.

Her eyes flicked to the sound of their voices, but she clearly looks exhausted and barely moves. There is clear use of accessory muscles of her neck when drawing in the air and her skin appears ashen grey, suggesting severe cyanosis. She manages to cough producing a very chesty sound.

Her response levels would be alert with a clear airway. Her breathing rate was raised from the text book 'normal' but for Mrs Underhill this was a daily occurrence. The attending paramedic decides to leave her on her O_2 and get a saturation probe on her finger while assessing her circulation, which produced a weak, thready and fast pulse of 120. The home O_2 cannula was swapped for an ambulance service nasal cannula that also had a built in end tidal CO_2 monitor. The driver, a student paramedic, places the 10 electrodes onto the patient for a 12-lead ECG while the attending paramedic takes a blood pressure reading.

Baseline observations following the primary survey are:

AVPU:	fully alert;
Airway:	open and clear of fluids or sputum;
Respiration rate:	24 bpm and regular with use of accessory muscles;
Pulse:	120 bpm, weak and thready;
BP:	102/61 mmHg (patient seated);

12 Lead ECG	showed no ST elevation on a sinus tachycardia;
End Tidal CO_2	was producing 35 mmHg;
Temperature:	37.9°C (slightly raised, but not significant);
Blood glucose:	normal at 6.4 mmol/L;
SpO_2:	below 90%. As this remains down to 87% after five minutes and there is evidence of cyanosis, high-flow O_2 is administered at 15 L per minute by a non-rebreathing mask and careful monitoring noted to ensure it is adjusted in line with any subsequent rise of SpO_2;

Glasgow Coma Scale: 15/15.

Oxygen saturation (SpO_2), 'the fifth vital sign' (along with pulse, blood pressure, temperature and respiratory rate) should be checked by pulse oximetry in all breathless and acutely ill patients and the inspired oxygen concentration should be recorded on the patient report form with the oximetry result. It is essential that with the change in mask used for O_2 delivery the patient is monitored continuously against respiratory effort.
General appearance is paler than normal with signs of fatigue.

The British Thoracic Society (1997) Guidelines on Oxygen state:

Treatment for COPD should be commenced using a 28% Venturi mask at 4 L/min in pre-hospital care with an initial target saturation of 88–92% pending urgent blood gas results. These patients should be treated as a high priority by emergency services and the oxygen dose should be reduced if the saturation exceeds 92%.

---

1   **What problems are highlighted above, in the baseline observations?**

A   This lady has a higher respiratory rate than we would expect which, as mentioned, might be relatively normal for her. It is essential that with the change in O_2 delivery the patient is monitored continuously against respiratory effort. The hypoxia present with Gladys also pushes her heart rate up, which may also be influenced by the anxiety of struggling to breathe. The blood pressure is low which might be **idiopathic** (if this is normal) or could be a sign of **hypovolaemia** if she is dehydrated or could be a sign of infection. It is important to consider this in patients with COPD as they are far more susceptible to respiratory tract infections such as bronchitis and pneumonia which can exacerbate their COPD symptoms. This suspicion is raised further in her mildly raised body temperature.

2   **What are the TIME CRITICAL features for this patient?**

A   • Severe hypoxia (87% O_2) which is unresponsive to O_2;
• Exhaustion and accessory muscle use in her breathing;
• Cyanosis (more severe than normal).

These all indicate that it is vital to transfer her to the nearest ED for more intensive management.

3 **What is the primary diagnosis at this stage in the proceedings?**

A COPD (Chronic Obstructive Pulmonary Disease) is a general term which covers many previously used clinical labels which are all presentations of a similar problem (e.g. chronic bronchitis, emphysema, chronic obstructive airways disease, and even some cases of chronic asthma).

COPD is a chronic, slowly progressive disorder characterized by airway obstruction which does not change markedly over several months. The impairment to the function of the lung is generally fixed but may be changed with the use of bronchodilator therapy. The primary cause is generally long-term smoking. Sadly, COPD causes significantly more morbidity and mortality than other limiting airflow situations.

4 **What would you expect to see on examination?**

A In COPD bilateral reduction in chest wall movement but no tracheal deviation. A normal percussion note is heard and normal vocal resonance. An expiratory **polyphonic wheeze** is heard with coarse crackles but expiration is prolonged. Patients often complain of a long-standing cough and regularly suffer with respiratory infections. Any symptoms can be exacerbated by cold weather and pollution. As the disease progresses, patients can experience severe breathlessness on simple tasks such as dressing so it is important to briefly assess their ability with daily tasks (are they finding themselves getting breathless while just sitting, can they complete a spoken sentence?) to establish their deterioration and need for hospital care.

Gladys already has a COPD diagnosis but you should be considering why she is still deteriorating for the sake of handover. The initial signs show that you suspect an underlying infection which is exacerbating her symptoms but you should rule out a cardiovascular component via ECG. Also you should question whether the patient has been taking their medication appropriately and is it in date. Gathering the medicines into a bag and bringing them to the ED assists all elements of the care to understand any **polypharmacy**. Inhalers are notoriously taken very badly and inhaled drugs do expire while having the risk of being faulty. In the elderly there is sometimes the risk of forgetting to take their drugs or taking the wrong dose.

It was clear from the supplementary questions that Gladys was now becoming more unwell at home and with the increased cyanosis, breathlessness reduced levels of activity and mobility it was no longer an option to leave her on home care and O_2. She was therefore transported to the nearest ED.

---

5 **What is the long-term care?**

A While there are treatments to control COPD and relieve the symptoms, they are at best palliative. On a worldwide scale it has been estimated that by the year 2020, COPD will be the fifth highest disease burden to society. The World Health Organization (WHO; Hurd 2000) estimates that in 2000, 2.74 million people died of COPD worldwide and that passive smoking is associated with a 10–43% increase in risk of COPD in adults. However, only 10–20% of heavy smokers actually go on to develop COPD, suggesting some level of genetic susceptibility. The British Thoracic Society (1997) state that the consultation rates in COPD are 2–4 times that for angina. This means that the disease burden is on the rise, especially with an ageing population and is something you are likely to see on a more regular basis.

6   **When should we reduce the high-flow oxygen? What about hypoxic drives?**

A   It has been said that while CO_2 is what influences respiration centrally, it is also thought that those with COPD tend to become less sensitive to CO_2 over time and gain a level of control from the relative hypoxia, hence why oxygen can be restricted. There has been some considerable debate about this, but the following are the recommended guidelines to follow along with your own sensible judgement. Use a 28% Venturi mask at 4 L/min and aim for an oxygen saturation of 88–92% for patients with risk of **hypercapnia** but this target range can be shifted to 94–98% if the $PaCO_2$ is normal (which you will be unable to record in the ambulance).

REFERENCES

British Thoracic Society (1997) Guidelines for the management of chronic obstructive pulmonary disease. *Thorax* 52 (Suppl. 5): S1–S32.

Hurd, S. (2000) The impact of COPD on lung health worldwide: epidemiology and incidence. *Chest* 117: S1–S4.

Crown Hotel

Case outline

A call is made from the Crown Hotel in central Edinburgh. The patient, a young Italian tourist, was experiencing sudden-onset chest pain that had woken her in the early hours of the morning. She had attempted to walk it off with a morning stroll in the street but had found that it was painful to walk and her chest pain and sudden dyspnoea were getting worse. She made it back to reception by taxi where the staff then called for an ambulance.

Marina, a 23 year old, had arrived recently from Naples and was here to improve her English. The crew were able to communicate with her via her friend, Antonia, who had a better understanding of English. Although the foyer was a public thoroughfare it was 6 am and no one was around except the hotel duty manager on reception.

Clearly alert, but in pain, particularly on inspiration, suggesting pleuritic pain, she was holding her chest and looked very anxious. The paramedic considered her a very young candidate for a heart condition, but worked through basics to eliminate false positives to establish the working diagnosis.

The baseline observations following the primary survey are:

AVPU:	alert
Airway:	clear and dry
Respiratory Rate:	30 bpm
Circulation:	142 bpm
Pupils:	PEARRL (Size 3)
Temperature:	37.8°C
Blood sugar:	4.9 mmol/L
BP:	94/54 mmHg
SpO$_2$:	88%
GCS:	15/15
General appearance:	slightly cyanosed lips and peripherals. She also was experiencing a minor cough.

On physical examination, **a pleural rub** was heard on **auscultation** in the upper part of her right lung. Further history from Antonia revealed Marina had flown in the day before and had been fit and well and was not being treated by any medications, even though she was feeling slightly warm, which was confirmed by the slightly raised

tympanic temperature measurement. She had not been drinking or taken any drugs; however she admitted to smoking 15 cigarettes per day and had done so for around five years. She also revealed that she has been prescribed a new oral contraceptive approximately two months previously.

1 **What is your working diagnosis?**

A Pulmonary embolism (PE) is the most likely diagnosis, which is a blockage of one of the arteries of the lung by an embolism, usually a thrombus. This obstructs the blood flow through the lungs and can result in pressure on the right side of the heart and leads to the symptoms and signs of chest pain. PE, along with deep vein thrombosis (DVT), is a condition that commonly occurs after a long-haul flight so must be considered in someone with a recent travel history. You must always consider the possibility of cardiac involvement in chest pain and remember that one of the causes of the appearances of an MI in young people is illicit drug (cocaine) use so you should attempt to rule this out with an ECG and detailed chest pain history. There may also be a congenital heart problem that is affecting her at such a young age and she might be unaware of a potential problem. Also consider that trauma can also cause chest pain, raised heart rate and breathing with a low blood pressure.

> **Classic Causes of PE Are**
> Extended travel (car, plane, train). Even prolonged bed rest. No research has yet defined what is meant by prolonged so although the patient has only flown from southern Italy, it still should be considered as prolonged immobilization.

2 **Why might this NOT be cardiac?**

A Cardiac pain generally arrives suddenly but is NOT aggravated or diminished by position of the patient or the breathing. In this case the patient is female and aged 23 which would place her in a very low risk group. An ECG should be carried out in the vehicle to clarify if there are ECG changes even if we thought this was linked to drug use. So while it is not ruled out, her risk is very low.

3 **How time critical is this situation?**

A Severe cases of PE can lead to sudden collapse, abnormal and falling blood pressure and sudden death (around 15% of all cases).

4 **So how can we be definitive with any diagnosis, with so many options?**

A Definitive diagnosis can only be truly found at the hospital based on the clinical findings and in combination with laboratory tests (such as the **D-dimer test**) and imaging studies, usually via **computer tomography (CT)** pulmonary angiography. Treatment is typically via **anticoagulant** medication, including **warfarin** or **heparin**. Severe cases have received thrombolytics such as tissue

> **Pulmonary embolism** (PE) is the third most common cardiovascular disease after acute ischemic syndromes and stroke and is the first cause of death in hospitalized patients older than 65 and the first cause of death in women during pregnancy (Pierluigi 2001).

plasminogen activator (tPA) or may require more aggressive surgical intervention such as pulmonary thrombectomy.

Therefore it is vital to make a fast transfer to the nearest E D and give a complete handover of the detailed history you have obtained with the significant details.

Treating Marina in pre-hospital care will be to give oxygen to counteract her cyanosis and raise her oxygen saturation. Communication to this young lady will be vital to overcome her fear and her pain. Her B P is quite low so it would be wise to act cautiously and use an alternative pain relief such as **Entonox** as it contains 50% O_2 but will have to be considered in proportion to her respiratory effort as it is self-administered. Morphine will lower her B P to a dangerous level.

Her heart rate remains raised with a low B P. Should it fall any further consider this to be suspicious and start an I V and give a 250 ml fluid challenge of sodium chloride 0.9%.

Without drawing attention to your concerns make sure your advanced airway kit is at hand and ready to use. Although prognosis is normally good (around 95% survival) some patients who have massive P E undiagnosed for one or two hours can collapse suddenly and a respiratory arrest may be the next step.

---

5   **What sort of unusual presentations should you look for in this patient?**

A   The patient might not always present with profound chest pain. They may simply be suffering with respiratory distress and signs of further emboli (e.g. thrombophlebitis or D V T).

Peripheral pulses may not always be felt and also be aware of respiratory problems when the O_2 saturation is undetectable. Some patients might simply present with profound cyanosis.

P E can also cause circulatory collapse in severe situations so you might see coronary involvement in the E C G (e.g. a sinus tachycardia or right bundle branch block). However, this makes ruling out cardiac causes very difficult, but still all points to the fact that the situation is critical and the patient should be transferred without delay.

6   **What are the risk factors for a PE?**

A   • Smoking;
• Oral contraceptive pill;
• **Coagulopathy**;
• Immobility (e.g. long flight).

7   **In what other circumstances might a PE occur?**

A   A pulmonary embolism is a blockage of an artery in the lung usually by a thromboemboli. It can be associated with a clot in the deep veins in the leg and so often seen alongside a D V T. It can also be a risk post-surgery due to the disruption of vascular supply which can send smaller clots into the bloodstream, so be aware of this complication if a patient tells you they have recently had any surgery.

8 **What is the outcome likely to be for this patient?**

A Outcome can be based on time of transfer and delay of patient calling the ambulance from the onset of symptoms. Also, the vessel affected can vary massively as to what tissue it supplies so extent of damage is unpredictable. A P E which is detected early and treated early will have a better outcome.

9 **Is there specific treatment for this patient?**

A The important supportive features in pre-hospital care are to monitor the heart rate and E C G for signs of cardiac deterioration and monitor the blood pressure, giving supportive fluid therapy.

Key learning points

- Get to know the local guidelines in place for treating a major P E with thrombolysis.
- There is a high mortality associated with the treatment, often occurring in the first hour of administration and the risks of haemorrhage are the critical issue.
- Provide supportive therapy and transfer to the nearest E D for further investigation.

REFERENCE

Pierluigi, P. (2001) Diagnosis and management of pulmonary embolism: a categorical teaching seminar presented at the European Association of Nuclear Medicine meeting in Naples, Italy.

Case outline

The crew is called to see an adult female who has collapsed on a city centre train with chest pain. On arrival, the crew can see the ambulance service rapid response unit (RRU) outside the Lime Street railway station, and decide to take the trolley-bed off the ambulance and place all the kit on it to take to the scene. It can be a long walk back from a platform to the street to get kit, especially in the crowds during rush hour.

1   **What would you take to the scene?**

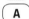

- Primary response bag (PRB);
- Oxygen therapy equipment;
- Paramedic bag and resuscitation drugs;
- Aspirator (portable);
- Orthopaedic scoop or rescue backboard;
- Securing straps for the above;
- Blankets for warmth and modesty.

They are all potentially useful; however, if you are a multiple responder then you may not wish to duplicate. Your service may have a minimum kit response that the RRU will have taken. It would be better not to duplicate, except for perhaps a defibrillator. Many public places have defibrillators and trained staff ready to use them, but you can't be certain that one has been taken to scene.

The station managers meet you at the entrance, which is very helpful as some large railway and underground stations can have multiple access points. Hopefully your Emergency Operations Centre (EOC) have given you a **rendezvous point (RVP)**, to speed up access and improve egress when you leave.

It takes you over five minutes from street to scene to negotiate the concourse and corridors and, as you enter the platform, you can see ahead of you an inexperienced paramedic from the RRU, who is known to you, attempting to intubate an adult women of early retirement age. Members of the railway staff are carrying out what appears to be effective resuscitation and an automated external defibrillator (AED) is attached to the patient's chest.

You are told by the first paramedic on scene that 'we have given one shock, still in VF, can't get a vein so trying to secure the airway'. Little is known about this lady at this point as she was travelling alone so you check to see if she has any ID on her or any **medic alert emblems** that would give you more information at this point.

2 **What are your priorities at this stage?**

A
- **Danger** – is it still safe to approach?
- **Response** – is there any response from the patient?
- **Airway** – is this patent and clear?
- **Breathing** – is she spontaneously breathing?
- **Circulation** – is there a pulse and if so is it adequate circulation to perfuse the patient?

You must establish that it is safe for you, and not assume that everyone else is on scene, so it must be. Fortunately the patient is away from the platform edge and the British Transport Police (BTP) and rail staff have got the small crowd held well away.

It is vital that you get briefed on arrival so that your team efforts are supportive for the patient.

> The resus council guidelines suggest that if a health professional witnesses out of hospital arrest, they should not delay defibrillation but if it is unwitnessed, they should give two minutes of CPR prior to initiating defibrillation (ERC 2010).

3 **What is the most important next action of the following, and why?**

A
- Intubation;
- Cannulation;
- Defibrillation;
- Cardiopulmonary resuscitation;
- Scoop and run to the nearest ED;
- Cardiac drugs.

Logically you'll say airway, breathing and circulation (ABC), but in fact intubation at this stage is only required if you cannot maintain the airway by manual methods of positioning and effective use of a BVM (bag valve mask). The most important thing is to maintain effective cardiac massage, therefore continue with quality cardiopulmonary resuscitation. This has proven to have the most effect in many studies in the past few years. Early defibrillation on a witnessed arrest is the second most useful.

Gaining an IV is very helpful to administer the adrenaline and amiodarone if the heart remains in defibrillator resistant VF. Placing double quantities of the cardiac drugs down the endotracheal tube is not advised and has no evidence of effectiveness.

> There is no evidence to support or refute the use of any specific airway in resuscitation so a laryngeal mask airway (LMA) is now commonly used. However, a tracheal intubation tube is perceived as optimal for maintaining the airway, known as 'the gold standard'.

Unless there is an overriding reason, such as multi-patients, it is best to work alongside the first paramedic. One of the crew should try to cannulate and support the compressions, while the other one should provide crichoid pressure to improve view of the vocal chords for the intubation. This is all done with high-quality CPR and defibrillation as the main priority.

Defibrillation

The recommended biphasic defibrillation energy is 150–200 J and any subsequent shocks at 150–360 J. In a monophasic defibrillator, the energy should be at 360 J for the first and all subsequent shocks.

You should move the patient to the nearest ED in the event of regaining spontaneous rhythm after ensuring the patient is stable or, if there is no further improvement, recognition of life extinct (ROLE) and move the patient to a mortuary or ED as per the local protocol (due to this occurring in a public place).

4   **What are the shockable rhythms?**

A   VF and pulseless VT are shockable rhythms. Non-shockable rhythms include pulseless electrical activity (PEA) or asystole and of course any palpable pulse.

5   **When do you give adrenaline to the patient?**

A   In PEA and asystole, give the first dose of 1 mg adrenaline 1:10000 as soon as IV access is achieved and then repeat every 3–5 minutes.

Adrenaline is given IV 1 mg in VT/VF and then repeated every 3–5 mins as long as VT/VF persists.

6   **Would you give any additional drugs?**

A   **Amiodarone** 300 mg (an anti-arrhythmic) is given when VT/VF has persisted for three shocks and then one repeated dose of 150 mg may be given in a recurrent or refractory VT/VF. This will be followed up with an infusion of 900 mg over 24 hours.

Lidocaine is sometimes considered for use when **amiodarone** is not available but in practice, it is rarely used. **Lidocaine** and **amiodarone**, when given together, increase risk of asystole.

7   **What are the four Hs and four Ts that need to be considered in a cardiac arrest and will they make any difference in a pre-hospital setting and why?**

A   On review, it is important to consider other reversible causes that you might or might not be able to deal with in the out-of-hospital setting but if possible you can also consider reversal or points to highlight on handover.

* Hypoxia: give high-flow oxygen via non-rebreath mask.
* Hypovolaemia: Ideally use the already established IV access; if none, place one large bore cannula, give saline and monitor BP.
* Hyperkalaemia, hypokalaemia, hypocalcaemia, acidaemia: go to hospital with any other metabolic disorders that cannot be accurately diagnosed on roadside.
* Hypothermia: thermal blankets to stabilize. You are not dead until warm and dead.
* Tension pneumothorax: decompress by needle thoracocentesis at the second intercostal space.

- Tamponade: transfer to E D. ECG obtained if possible.
- Toxic substances: gain as much information as you can from site and transfer to E D.
- Thromboembolism (pulmonary embolus/coronary thrombosis): ECG confirmed ST elevation in coronary thrombosis – transfer to local angioplasty service. If unconfirmed, send to nearest E D.

8   How long are you going to stay on the platform?

A   Public place or at home, resus is going to be better here on a firm platform than on a moving trolley-bed in corridors and escalators or even in the back of the ambulance.

When you have completed four shocks of C PR then it is advisable to review where you are at and what else you can do, whether that is staying on the platform or beginning to transfer the patient to hospital. If a pulse returns at any point, initiate post-resuscitation care.

9   What is the standard post-resuscitation care pathway?

A   • In hospital, a patient at this point would be transferred to **ITU** or **CCU**.
- The out-of-hospital aims at this point would be to maintain A BC and continue monitoring for deterioration.

Pre-hospital cooling might also be considered in some areas of the U K in a post-V F arrest, cooling to 32–34°C for 12–24 hours as temperatures above 37°C are associated with poor neurological outcomes. Not all patients will qualify for the cooling therapy criteria. Many trials are ongoing.

Airway and breathing

Ensure tracheal intubation is considered to maintain the optimum airway and control of ventilation (SpO$_2$ > 95%), close monitoring of end tidal CO$_2$ rising from 12 mmHg which you would see during cardiac arrest to aim to return to normal values of 35–45 mmHg, you are likely to see a value of about 24 mmHg after return of circulation.

Circulation

Circulation might still be unstable at this point so monitor B P closely. Fluids given to restore hypovolaemia and hypotension can help to stabilize at this point. Some experts advocate stabilizing for around 10 minutes on scene when you have a ROSC, prior to loading and heading for the nearest appropriate E D. This is still a controversial action, with other experts advocating load and go asap on ROSC.

Examine the neurological system for any early signs of problems and also measure the blood glucose to rule this out in case of deterioration of condition.

REFERENCE

European Resuscitation Council (E RC) (2010) Resuscitation Guidelines: Adult Advanced Life Support. Available at: http://www.resus.org.uk/pages/als.pdf

Case outline

The paramedic and her student paramedic are starting New Year's Day at 6 am on the early shift. First call of the day is from a print worker heading home after the night shift who had found a young man in his late teens huddled up in a shop doorway.

Cautious approaches are always required and you may well hope they are just sleeping off whatever they have taken. People do not like being wakened in the early hours when it's cold and damp from overnight rain. There was no response to the introductions, and no response to a very gentle touch on the patient's shoulder with a friendly, 'come on mate, wake up'. With a limited sluggish response it became necessary to be more firm with the assessments of consciousness and it was clear this guy was really out of it, smelling of stale vomit and old alcohol.

First thing to check is that he has a patent airway and is sufficiently 'with it', before you can start thinking of alternative future destinations. Sleeping rough after a heavy night is not a major priority to most of the local residents on any big city streets. He wasn't causing offence; if anything he was not cooperating with the crew, waking up and telling them to 'foxtrot oscar'.

---

1 **What would you do?**

1 Call the police, and let him sleep it off in a police cell.
2 Put him in the ambulance and take him to the nearest ED and let them greet the new year with a fresh drunk to monitor.
3 Continue to assess him to see if he's OK and if so leave him to sleep it off in the street and allow him to make his way 'home' later on.

A (1) Police are dealing with assault, drunkenness and multiple other problems in the early hours of New Year's Day. While it is not the police's responsibility to look after drunks, when a patient is uncooperative, unreasonably abusive or you suspect a need for the police to be involved, call them for assistance. You would be unlikely to require the police in this case though.

(2) The ED will have had the night from hell. In a normal day 35% of all patients presenting to the ED are alcohol related, with it doubling on Friday and Saturday evenings. New Year's Eve has been known to be as high as 90% drink related, which costs the NHS around £2bn a year. The Department of Health estimates that one million people were admitted to hospital due to alcohol-related harm in England in 2008–9, which is not surprising with alcohol consumption up 50% since 1970, particularly in the age group under 24.

(3) Alcohol masks symptoms and so it might be wise to continue the assessments as you are left responsible for the patient's treatment. So this is our best option.

The patient's general baseline observations are:

Airway: clear and dry (dehydrated) but with obnoxious smelling breath;
Breathing: is shallow at 12 bpm;
Circulation: pulse barely detectable at 40 bpm;
SpO$_2$:   monitor shows error, probably due to lack of peripheral circulation;
Temperature: recorded at 34°C. This might be inaccurate as tympanic thermometers are not particularly accurate on the very low scales, but are acceptable for pre-hospital care for the majority of patients seen in the UK (see Table 7.1);
BM: 6.2 mmol/L. It is worth double-checking we don't have an underlying diabetic who is cold and drunk. It is also worth noting that pre-hospital diagnostic equipment is prone to errors in low temperature.

---

2   **What observations are causes for concern?**

A   Bradycardia (defined as <60 bpm) suggests something more sinister:

- Bradycardia can occur as part of the effects of ageing on the heart or after a heart attack due to the damage to its conducting ability.
- Sick-sinus syndrome covers a range of problems involving a reduction in the number of beats initiated by the heart and heart block. A number of heart problems are involved in chronic bradycardia.
- There are also a number of non-cardiac causes related to electrolyte and endocrine imbalance.
- Also consider side effects from drug use (or abuse), especially when found the 'morning after the night before' and more common in a younger age group (although this isn't a blanket rule).

Table 7.1   Body temperature classification

Temperature classification	Core (rectal, oesophageal)
Hyperpyrexia	>40.0–41.5°C
Hyperthermia	>38.4–39.9°C
Fever	>37.5–38.3°C
Normal	36.5–37.5°C
Hypothermia	<35.0°C
Mild	32–35°C
Moderate	28–32°C
Severe	20–28°C
Profound	<20°C

- Although 40 is very low, a resting heart rate <60 is quite common among athletes and might be normal in a patient in their late teens.

> The patient is also mildly hypothermic and, along with the bradycardia, you should be concerned for the patient's condition. Be aware that the patient is likely to be **hypoperfused**, confirmed further by lack of peripheral circulation, risking **ischaemic** damage to vital organs such as the heart and kidneys. You can also check peripheral pulses to further assess this.

3 **What classic symptoms would you expect to see with hypothermia?**

A A range of symptoms occurs in hypothermia. Starting with the initial symptoms, vasocon-striction leads to a pale complexion and cold peripheries. The **hypothalamus** then stimulates shivering (to aid heat production) but this diminishes as the patient's core temperature comes to about 30–32°C. Neurological signs include muddled thinking, confusion and reduced co-ordination. At the extreme end of hypothermia, the patient's confusion and loss of thermo-regulation leads to paradoxical undressing, removing clothing as the body vasodilates and sends blood to warm the peripheries. Other non-specific signs include a slow weak pulse, pupil dilation and reduced respiratory rate.

4 **What is a clear definition of hypothermia?**

A Hypothermia is when the body's core temperature is lowered due to exposure to cold, gener-ally considered to be 35°C or less. The symptoms vary and also depend on the stage of the hypothermia. This patient is objectively mildly hypothermic but his symptoms suggest a more marked hypothermia with confusion and reduced consciousness. Considering his alcohol intake, this subjective measurement is more difficult.

5 **Who is at risk of hypothermia?**

A The very young and elderly have altered **thermoregulatory** mechanisms and so do not always react in a normal way to cold weather. As in this case, alcohol and drug use dampen the reaction to cold environments. Also consider that those living in colder environments such as the homeless or people unable to afford to heat their home, are at considerable risk of hypo-thermia and associated health risks of prolonged exposure to the cold, such as increased incidence of viral and bacterial infections.

> The crew have lifted him on to the trolley and got him into the slightly warmer ambu-lance. The crew are concerned about the mild hypothermia and make the decision the patient will need warming slowly at hospital. Alcohol has numbed his senses and thinned his blood; he probably wasn't even aware of how cold he was and still is, although he is slowly sobering up and starting to shiver.

6   **What is your management en route to hospital?**

A   The first thing is to remove the patient from the cold wet environment and insulate them from the cold wind that is blowing. This is known as passive rewarming. Lay an unconscious or semiconscious victim face up and wrap in blankets. Treat the victim for shock and transport to the nearest medical facilities as quickly as possible.

> Stage two will occur when in the care of the ED with a variety of strategies. Warm water immersion, heated blankets, warm objects, radiant heaters and forced air. These are all known as active external rewarming.
>
> However, there is an important phenomenon known as 'after drop': as initial active external rewarming leads to peripheral vasodilation (BP drops) cold blood from dilated peripheral vessels carries high **lactic acid** levels to core vessels. This cold **acidotic** blood causes drop in core temp and provokes serious **arrhythmias**. This is why it is vital that it occurs in hospital where they can monitor the patient more easily and intervene where necessary.

Key learning points

- Recognize the signs and symptoms of hypothermia and be careful not to miss them if found alongside other comorbidities.
- Be aware of the risks of 'after drop' during rewarming and how this impacts your management of the patient en route to hospital.

Case outline

Jim Beko, a 67-year-old man from Reading, called his **General Practitioner (GP)** early in the morning stating he had noticed blood in his urine following surgery six weeks before for his benign **prostatic hypertrophy**. As the GP was in the middle of surgery Jim spoke with the receptionist and she advised him to call NHS Direct. From the description of his symptoms and considering his past medical history, they suggested an ambulance was called so that he could be more closely assessed for risk of further deterioration.

On arrival at his terraced home, one crew member remembered being called out to the house about a year before for a **hypoglycaemic** episode in an elderly diabetic gentleman. Today the incident was dispatched to them as male adult bleeding into his urine (haematuria). The attendant was considering if his previous call might be connected to this one.

After around two minutes delay the front door was finally opened by a frail man who looked quite unwell. His movements were slow and lethargic and so the crew got him to sit on the chair in the hall.

He tells the ambulance crew that he hasn't felt very well the past five or six days. He says that he is suffering with some back, side and groin pain and has noticed an increased urgency and burning with urination. He noticed that his urine has a pink tinge *yesterday* but it has got worse overnight and now looks like blood (bright red). He now feels nauseous and has vomited once this morning and also has quite profound diarrhoea which has left him pale, lethargic and a little breathless. Mr Beko's catheter was removed four weeks ago on a regular check-up at the outpatients. He is very apologetic for calling the ambulance, and explains he tried to talk to his GP and NHS Direct but they had suggested he phoned 999. He says he is often unwell and isn't sure why everyone is so worried about him, he just wanted to check the symptoms were normal with his GP.

Further questioning is undertaken while baseline observations are gathered. His medical problems include **hypertension** for the past year and type II diabetes for the last five years. Last year he was treated for **gout** after he'd reported a painful left **metatarsal-phalangeal** joint. The GP had prescribed **allopurinol** and **colchicine**. His gout pain is pretty much resolved.

The baseline observations following the primary survey are:

Airway: clear and dry, no odour;
Breathing: slightly raised at 24 bpm;

Circulation: 120 bpm;
BP: 120/76 mmHg (patient states that is lower than his normal reading);
SpO$_2$:   94% on air;
Temperature: 38.4°C by tympanic (signs of a slight fever);
BM: 5.8 mmol/L;
Pain score: pain is moderate and classed as 6 out of 10.

The lowered oxygen saturation of 94% triggers the attendant to give O$_2$ via an adult nasal cannula at 24% on 2 L a minute.

The crew monitor these baseline observations for any further changes while conducting further physical examination. The patient doesn't appear to be **time critical** so a secondary survey is conducted on Jim inside the house. His abdomen is sore to palpation, partly from vomiting which is now non-productive, and he claims to be moderately bloated. His back and sides are still quite tender and he remains a pale grey colour.

Medications on his bedside cabinet, which he has gathered before the arrival of the ambulance, include:

- **Ramipril** 2.5 mg every morning (started seven months ago);
- **Gliclazide** 40 mg twice daily;
- **Allopurinol** 400 mg once daily;
- **Colchicine** 2 mg once daily;
- **Ranitidine** 150 mg twice daily.

1   **How is this patient's medical history related to his current complaint?**

A   Type II diabetes is related to microvascular disease, which leads to diabetic **nephropathy**. Signs of diabetic nephropathy are **oedema**, generalized itching and vomiting, though it can also be **asymptomatic** in its early stages. Urine analysis would be needed for diagnosis and so would require either hospital admission if unwell or GP investigation. This however doesn't explain fully all of his symptoms. It is generally thought that microscopic blood in the urine is related to the kidneys and visible blood is related to damage to the bladder and urinary tract, such as infection, inflammation and **carcinoma**. It also has to be considered that this patient is suffering from complications of his **prostate** surgery such as trauma from the urinary catheter or infection.

You would not be expected to know what the problem is at this point but be aware of the general causes of blood in the urine and use that to guide your history taking, taking into account relevant medical conditions and symptoms/signs in the patient. You would of course ideally (if in your scope of practice) want to take a urine dipstick (indicating infection, glucose etc.) wherever you transfer the patient to.

2   **What are the primary causes of blood in the urine (haematuria)?**

A   Haematuria can be described as painful or painless, helping to further differentiate a cause. A few common examples are given below. Remember that no presenting complaint is absolute and that each one of these can present differently.

Painless:

- Tumours (kidneys, ureter, bladder or prostate);
- Renovascular disease;
- Glomerulonephritis;
- Coagulation disorders.

Painful:

- Urinary tract infection (UTI);
- Renal calculi/stones causing obstruction (these are extremely painful).

The patient doesn't complain of any pain on urinating so it is less likely to be a full UTI or obstruction. However, given recent prostate surgery, it could still be a UTI (commonly caused by indwelling urinary catheters in the hospital setting). Blood could also be from his prostate, either due to trauma or a tumour. Prostatitis (infection of the prostate) can also present with haematuria.

The message here is that the diagnosis is very unclear and essentially requires further investigations that are not possible in the primary care setting.

3 **Should the crew call the GP to visit after surgery or would it be wiser to take Mr Beko to the nearest hospital and for what reason?**

A Given his medical problems and recent surgery, you might feel it is safe to assume that he should be taken to the GP where his symptoms can be easily assessed. However, kidney problems are often a complicated issue to tackle and the GP may feel more comfortable with him seeing a renal specialist at the hospital where the surgery was carried out. He also has been acutely unwell and may require immediate treatment that the GP cannot give.

4 **As the ambulance is not a taxi service, should Mr Beko make his own way there?**

A Again, probably not. It would be wiser for Jim to be in hospital where analysis of his blood and other investigations are used to monitor his progress and where medical staff would be more likely to have an idea of the cause of his symptoms. He is clearly weak and his condition could deteriorate at any time. Given that he is also alone at home, it is safer to take him straight to the hospital once your history and examination is complete. He is also complaining of pain (score of 6) so he will need analgesia.

5 **If Mr Beko had presented post-surgically with reduced urination, oedema and an acutely unwell condition (malaise, vomiting), how would your differential diagnosis have changed?**

A Reduced urination can be caused by several factors:

1 Lack of urine production: renal failure, severe dehydration.
2 Obstruction to urination: enlarged prostate, renal calculi obstructing the bladder, neurological problem affecting the opening of the valves in the bladder controlling urine flow.

Given that he is still urinating this makes complete obstruction by stone or neurological problem unlikely. The most likely explanation here is as a result of reduced urine production (i.e. failure of the kidneys).

Acute renal failure is now referred to as acute kidney injury. Causes of this are divided up into the following categories:

- Pre-renal: reduced blood flow (severe hypotension, dehydration/hypovolaemia or renovascular disease). This results in hypoperfusion of the kidneys and a reduced glomerular filtration rate.
- Intrinsic (in the kidney): damage to the glomeruli (glomerulonephritis), tubules (acute tubular necrosis) or interstitial disease (interstitial nephritis).
- Post-renal: malignancy or renal stone causing obstruction.

6   **What is the most likely diagnosis in this patient given his medical history of diabetes and hypertension?**

A   Diabetes can give rise to vascular disease and **nephropathy**, which would be a pre-renal cause of this gentleman's renal failure. Given its rapid onset you would suspect an acute kidney injury due to renovascular disease. He may also be dehydrated which is compounding his renal problems so a fluid challenge of 250 ml sodium chloride 0.9% should be considered.

> Acute kidney injury has a rapid onset time, peaking at less than 48 hours from the start.

7   **How would you manage an acute kidney injury?**

A   Management depends on the underlying cause so ensuring the patient is in a stable condition (airway clear, oxygen therapy, etc.) should be the focus. Fluid resuscitation can be difficult in these patients and should be carried out with extreme caution. Too much fluid could result in pulmonary oedema and require additional diuretic therapy. Avoid **colloid** fluids as they might increase **plasma protein** levels.

Acute kidney injury causes **metabolic acidosis** and **hyperkalaemia** (the ED will measure **serum potassium** and treat if >6 mmol). Severe changes in potassium levels can give ECG changes and risks arrhythmias. If there is hyperkalaemia, avoid giving fluids containing high levels of potassium.

Management of renal patients is complex and especially in the pre-hospital setting where a diagnosis is generally not clear. Immediate transfer to hospital where a diagnosis can be made and the patient closely monitored is the most important aspect.

Key learning points

- You are not expected to be an expert in renal disease and the diagnosis is unlikely to be clear in a pre-hospital setting.
- Use the medical history to point you in the right direction and closely monitor the patient throughout your management.
- Rapid transfer should occur in any patient who is acutely unwell or unstable.

Case outline

A police car making contact with a pedestrian is unlikely to be a minor call given the speeds they might be required to drive in an emergency.

The police traffic car, now stationary, with a tell-tale bull's-eyed front windscreen and a second police car in attendance at the rear, further up the hill forming a fend-off position to protect the scene and the patient. The patient is lying on his back, on the ground around 2 m in front of the bonnet, of the first police car.

Initial thinking

- Is it safe?
- Is this person on the ground the only patient, was anybody else hurt?
- How are the police officers who have been directly involved in the collision?

Following confirmation that it is safe to proceed, it is the job of the first paramedic to appropriately triage the patients on the scene and treat the most life threatening first so this initial survey is an important step. There is only one patient involved and the police state no one else was involved in the incident so you prepare to approach the patient to assess the condition.

The paramedics **mobile data terminal (MDT)** in the RRU, used to interface information to ambulance crews has stated that an ambulance resource was dispatched and should be joining the scene in around four to five minutes. That is not long but can be a lifetime if the patient is **red flagged**, (i.e. time dependant and critical).

The patient is lying quite still with his eyes closed. The gentleman has experienced a 30 mph impact off the front of the car and a hard landing on the tarmac, 2 m from the grill. Police state he has not moved since the impact and has remained unconscious.

A bystander who is a keen first aider and a local health care assistant offers their help and quickly has the patient's head clamped between her two hands to stop any movement of the head and neck. The **mechanism of injury** (i.e. the windscreen damage, the dented bonnet and the testimony of the police) is a clear indication of a suspected c-spine injury.

Initial findings

AVPU: unconscious throughout pre-hospital care.

Catastrophic haemorrhage: nothing obvious on first glance, however there is obvious bleeding from the back of the head as it is now seeping on to the road. No obvious fluids from nose and ears are considered a positive sign.

Airway: clear, with a small non-bleeding cut lip; perhaps the patient bit their lip on impact. An oropharyngeal airway is sized from the incisors to the angle of the jaw and placed. Avoid NP airways with head injuries.

Breathing: 14 bpm bilateral chest rise with no obvious flail segments.

Circulation: full and bounding at 56 beats per minute.

BP: 105/58 mmHg.

SpO$_2$: 96% on air (98% on oxygen).

Pupils: equal but larger than normal at 6 mm and very sluggish to react.

BM: 6.5 mmol/L.

Temp: 36.9°C.

1 **Why use an oropharangeal airway?**

A The oropharangeal airway (sometimes referred to as the Guedel airway) is inserted using the 'chin lift' or 'jaw thrust' technique (in case of c-spine injury) and ensuring the airway is clear of debris and secretions. It is often the 'go-to airway' until a more definitive option is decided on depending on the patient's state. It is also better tolerated by patients who are semi-conscious as other options will be uncomfortable.

Oropharangeal airways are indicated in any patient with a reduced GCS (mental state assessment) with the patient being unconscious. Also place the airway if there is damage to the mouth e.g. loss of teeth. A nasopharyngeal airway (NPA) is always avoided with possible head injuries in case of base of skull fractures as this could create further complications.

2 **What are the classical symptoms of a head injury?**

A Symptoms in head injury can vary greatly and while some patients have obvious signs straight away, others may have no symptoms at the time of injury and go into serious deterioration after what is sometimes termed a '**lucid interval**'. This can be because signs only show as the bleeding or swelling presses on part of the brain or compresses neurovascular structures. The reason swelling and bleeding cause such severe symptoms in the brain are that the skull will not expand to accommodate the increasing volume and so the pressure increases.

The first symptoms will therefore be as a result of swelling and include headache, confusion, reduced consciousness and sometimes nausea and vomiting. The patient's conscious-ness will then continue to drop until they are unresponsive. You might see widened pupils at this point.

A long-term complication of the increased pressure from head injuries is **herniation** of the brain stem causing coma and death, usually two or three days after the accident. This is why bleeds into the brain are often treated by surgical intervention to relieve the pressure.

Symptoms suggestive of serious pathology include:

- observed changes in pupil's size, shape or unequal sizing;
- fracture of the skull with swelling at the site of injury;
- B P rise from normal reading (part of **Cushing's triad**);
- heart rate reduced (part of **Cushing's triad**);
- increasing confusion/drowsiness or loss of consciousness;
- respiratory rate reduced (part of **Cushing's triad**).

Regularly check the patient's vital signs for hypoxia and hypotension, two causes of secondary injury to the brain and other organs.

3 **What does the primary survey need to include?**

A (a) The c-spine must be continually stabilized (currently done by the H C A) but will require a cervical collar and you need to consider the possibility of vertebral fracture when opening the airway or moving the patient.

(b) An oropharangeal airway has already been placed but be prepared to put in a laryngeal mask airway or perform endotracheal intubation if the oropharangeal airway is contraindicated or if the patient's oxygen saturation is not improving with the current airway option. Ensure adequate oxygenation by giving the patient high-flow oxygen via a non-rebreathing mask.

(c) Assess circulation and watch for dropping blood pressure which might indicate hypovol-aemia due to the bleeding (internally or externally) but is not likely to be linked to the current head injury. Gain venous access by placing a large-bore cannula in both arms. The patient may require fluids to replace his blood volume being lost due to the injuries sustained. Cannulas will also be useful should a blood transfusion be required on entry to hospital and to prevent delay in starting the patient on more fluids on arrival.

(d) Assess and reassess the patient's level of consciousness using the **Glasgow Coma Scale** and assess pupil size, shape and reactivity.

The ambulance arrives just as the R R U paramedic is starting a quick neck-to-knees assessment. This situation is time critical and this patient needs moving on to hospital. He is breathing, although the rate is slower at 14 than the crew would really like, but both lungs are inflating. There are no obvious signs of fractures of ribs or pelvis; however, the left leg is very swollen on the mid thigh (compared to his right) and is considered to be fractured until otherwise proven by X-ray at the hospital. The arriving crew place a non-rebreather oxygen mask on the patient followed by gathering a secondary set of observations: blood pressure, a glucose reading and a tympanic temperature. They are also briefed on the state of play and it is decided that the patient should be **scooped up** by an orthopaedic stretcher and lifted on to the rescue board. One crew member, with the help of a police officer, gathers the trolley from the ambulance while the other two paramedics apply a collar and take over the head support from the HCA.

4 **What order are the straps secured on the long rescue board and why?**

A 1 With extra ambulance staff, police and an HCA it is possible to **log roll** the patient on to the board. Lowering an orthopaedic stretcher can reduce unnecessary movement.

2 Maintaining a good grip of the head, the patient is centralized upon the board while the straps are applied, initially just loosely.

3 The chest straps are secured first. This is to ensure the bulk of the body is properly held in position first. When a patient is conscious ask them to take a deep breath prior to final tightening; with an unconscious patient try to ensure they are tightened on the inspiratory cycle.

4 Leg straps and figure of eight around the ankles are secured next.

5 Finally the head blocks either side of the patient's head are secured. It is important to place the chin and forehead straps in position and secure either side in unison to stop pulling the head to left or right.

> The patient is then safe to remove and can be quickly re-assessed in the rear of the ambulance by two of the paramedics whilst the other places an alert call to the local ED which fortunately happens to be at a hospital with a specialist neurological and head injury unit. The patient remains unconscious en route but all baseline observations are currently stable.

Secondary observations

AVPU:	unconscious;
Catastrophic haemorrhage:	still nothing obvious;
Airway:	remains clear;
Breathing:	14 bpm;
Circulation:	56 bpm;
BP:	105/58 mmHg;
SpO$_2$:	96% on air (98% on oxygen);
Pupils:	equal and sluggish reaction at 6 mm;
BM:	6.5 mmol/L;
Temp:	36.9°C.

5 **How common are head injuries?**

A Traumatic head injuries are a leading cause of death and disability in children and young adults, with around 700,000 people per year attending hospital emergency departments with a head injury in England and Wales. They commonly occur during a fall, an assault or road traffic collisions. Falls are the most common cause and tend to affect those at the extreme ends of age (i.e. children and the elderly). Alcohol might be involved in up to 65% of adult head injuries.

Very few patient will develop serious complications as a result of head injury. The rate of death after a head injury is still 0.2% so closely monitor the patient for deterioration and be prepared for a rapid transfer should this occur.

6 **What types of brain injury can occur?**

A **Localized:** cerebral contusions, skull fracture or haematoma as a result of direct trauma.

Diffuse: diffuse axonal injury following high-impact shear force to the body such as a road traffic collision. These are more severe and often lead to coma or persistent vegetative state.

These two types of injury can occur separately or at the same time, depending on the mode of injury.

Admission to hospital

The following are inclusion criteria for admission to hospital following a head injury:

* New, clinically significant abnormalities on imaging.
* Not returned to Glasgow Coma Scale (GCS) equal to 15 after investigations.
* Continuing worrying signs (e.g. persistent vomiting, severe headaches).

Key learning points

* Take note of any information you receive about the accident. The ED are likely to want to know some information about speed of impact, vehicle type and how far the patient was thrown which will help to give an estimation of the severity of the incident and possible internal damage.
* Monitor closely for the signs of hypoxia and hypotension which can lead to secondary damage to the brain and other organs.

Fast and furious

Case outline

Mr Jim Smith is a 64-year-old Caucasian man, whose wife called for an ambulance at just after 2 pm when he collapsed while gardening. On arrival, the ambulance crew finds the patient lying on his side on the garden patio. On initial assessment, he is conscious but unresponsive to questioning and so a history is taken from Mrs Smith while they examine the patient. She alludes that her husband very suddenly slumped to his knees and fell to the ground around 15 minutes before as they were walking back towards the house. His face looked droopy and she has been unable to understand his speech and he stopped answering her questions. She called for an ambulance and since then hasn't moved him and he is in the same condition as he was when he collapsed.

On further questioning of his wife, the paramedic crew discover that the patient had not been unconscious at all, had no obvious **seizure**, no episode of incontinence and no trauma prior to this incident. The patient had been feeling perfectly well despite his diabetes and was in no pain and had not complained of a headache. He had never experienced anything like this before.

Baseline observations

Response:	alert;
Airway:	open and clear;
Breathing:	16 bpm regular;
Circulation:	72 bpm and irregular;
	BP is 152/96 mmHg;
Disability:	conscious but drowsy;
	mini-neurological assessment conducted;
	Glasgow Coma Scale = 12/15 (moderate);
	general appearance (pale, drowsy), no MedicAlert bracelet.
Blood glucose:	slightly above normal at 7.9 mmol/L;
Temperature:	36.9°C.

Oxygen not used as this is not recommended at this point unless the patient is hypoxic.

1 **What is your current basic differential diagnosis?**

- elderly fall – hypotension, AF, MI (also consider a silent MI with Mr Smith's diabetic history);
- biochemical – hypoglycaemic;

- space-occupying lesion (abscess, tumour, haemorrhage);
- stroke;
- epilepsy.

A   Given the initial signs and symptoms, stroke is certainly the most likely with the information to hand and will be a good place to commence the rest of the assessments. Mr Smith is diabetic and so the crew will need to double-check that as they progress the assessments.

2   **What are the main subtypes that should be considered?**

A   **Transient Ischaemic Attack (TIA)** gives the same symptoms as a stroke but will resolve within 24 hours with no lasting damage. TIAs can cause any pattern of neurological dysfunction. They are thromboembolic in origin (microemboli) and pose a major risk factor for a subsequent disabling stroke. Strokes usually occur with a sudden onset but can have stepwise onset over several hours.

Ischaemic stroke (80–85%). These are common in an **arteriopath**. Usually an arterial embolus from a distant site (from carotid, vertebral or basilar arteries) or thrombosis of arteries, both causing infarction of the brain tissue supplied. Air and fat emboli, while uncommon, must also be considered.

Haemorrhagic stroke (15–20%). These are more common when the patient is long-term hypertensive, on anticoagulant treatment and is often preceded by a severe headache. Can be an intracerebral or subarachnoid haemorrhage but also can be the result of a Charcot-Bouchard aneurysm.

> **Charcot-Bouchard aneurysm**
> Microaneurysms of the brain vasculature, associated with chronic hypertension.

3   **What are the major risk factors that could increase the chances of suffering a stroke?**

A   The thromboembolic risks are commonly smoking, significant alcohol intake, sedentary life-style and a high Body Mass Index (BMI). Diabetes mellitus, atrial fibrillation, previous MI, high cholesterol, high blood pressure, previous TIA and peripheral vascular disease will also increase the risk. Rarer causes (unusual situations) include **anticardiolipin** or **lupus antico-agulant antibodies**, which should be considered in young patients as should coagulopathies (e.g. **thrombophilia**).

Endocarditis can also present with a thromboembolic stroke. Oral contraceptive pill (containing oestrogen) can predispose to strokes when combined with other uncontrolled risk factors. Drug abuse in illicit substances, such as cocaine, must also be considered as they are potent vasoconstrictors. Haemorrhagic risks often include hypertension, a genetic predisposition to aneurysms, anticoagulant and antiplatelet therapy and bleeding disorders.

> Mr Smith is currently on several types of medication, one for his cholesterol, an aspirin tablet and two blood pressure tablets, although his wife admits he's stopped taking one of his blood pressure tablets because he didn't like the side effects. His wife tells the crew that her husband has been told by the GP in the past that he has high cholesterol and high blood pressure but he takes tablets for them so must be fine. He also has an irregular heartbeat, but has had no other heart disease. He has recently been diagnosed with diabetes and has been trying to control this by dieting and is on tablets but does not take insulin.

Mr Smith has been a long-term smoker who smokes 20 cigarettes per day and has done for 40 years. He drinks about two pints (4 units) of beer each night. He is obese with a Body Mass Index (BMI) of about 31. His wife has been pleading with him to change his ways with his recently discovered diabetes, but Mr Smith has struggled to adapt.

4 **What are the possible classes of blood pressure medication, their mode of action and what side effects are common with each?**

A 1 **ACE inhibitors** reduce **angiotensin II** production (a potent vasoconstrictor) and so act to widen the blood vessels. Side effects include profound hypotension and also **bradykinin** build-up (due to reduced degradation) causing a persistent cough. Angiotensin receptor blockers (e.g. losartan) block angiotensin II receptors so have similar affects as ACE inhibitors but without bradykinin and there is no cough induced. They are usually given to patients who are unable to tolerate the ACE inhibitors.

2 **Beta-blockers** (e.g. **atenolol**): selective B_1 receptor agonist (cardioselective) works by inducing bradycardia and reducing the workload on the heart. Side effects can include bronchospasm (this drug is often avoided in asthma and COPD sufferers) and cold extremities.

3 **Calcium channel blockers** (e.g. **amlodipine**) have a negative inotropic effect on the myocardium to reduce the force of contraction. They also have a negative chronotropic effect, useful in reducing heart rate in atrial fibrillation and flutter.

4 **Diuretics**: there are two main subtypes of diuretics (or 'water tablets'). Loop diuretics (e.g. **spironolactone**) inhibit reabsorption of sodium and chloride ions in the 'loop of Henle' preventing the reabsorption of water. They are usually used in combination with other blood pressure-lowering drugs. Side effects include electrolyte imbalance (**hyponatraemia** and **hypokalaemia**) and postural hypotension. Thiazide diuretics (e.g. **bendroflumethiazide**) inhibit reabsorption of sodium and chloride ions in distal convoluted tubules to increase water excretion. They can cause increased serum cholesterol levels, hypokalaemia and **hyperuricaemia** (thereby precipitating gout).

> **Medications**
> Ask the patient (or relative in this case) to find the list of medications/prescription list or, if available, bring the drugs with you to the hospital. This will save hospital staff and patients precious time on clerking in if all drugs are together and available.

5 **Is this likely to be an ischaemic or haemorrhagic stroke?**

A His hypertension history and possible use of anticoagulants (for atrial fibrillation) provides a risk for haemorrhagic stroke but the lack of headache lessens this likelihood. However, his history is that of an arteriopath (increased risk of **atheromatous** plaques due to known risk factors) and so suggests that the root cause is ischaemic.

On examination, Mr Smith's face appears droopy on the right-hand side and has reduced movement on that side, when asked to smile. He is unable to lift his right arm, unable to grip with his right hand when asked and has reduced strength in his right leg. His left-hand side is of normal strength. Both pupils are equal and reactive to light (size 4).

Arteriopath
A patient prone to developing cardiovascular disease and is at risk due to various genetic and environmental factors (e.g. ethnicity, smoking, hypertension, hypercholesterolaemia).

6 **Based on the examination and current findings, what is your final diagnosis?**

A A left-sided middle cerebral arterial thromboembolism due to the nature of the contralateral motor deficit. The location is always more difficult to define due to the nature of the collateral blood supply of the brain. It is likely to be anterior/central in location due to the involvement of facial muscles and the expressive **aphasia**.

7 **What would be your management plan at this point?**

A Once you have decided on the potential diagnosis, it is important to move the patient quickly to the nearest hyperacute stroke unit (HASU), if available, in the semi-recumbent position (as this patient is still conscious and assuming the patient doesn't have a fracture as a result of the fall). Send a Pre-hospital Alert Message (Blue Call) stating that the patient is FAST positive/suspected acute stroke to ensure that the patient receives appropriate thrombolysis (often alteplase). Encourage an informant (friend or relative present) to accompany the patient as they will be helpful in completing the history at the hospital. If SpO_2 levels fall then consider oxygen to maintain saturation of more than 95% and ensure that the

Anyone with continuing neurological signs when first assessed should be assumed to have had a stroke.

blood glucose is at a normal level. If glucose level is low at <3.0 mmol/L, administer dextrose (100 ml 10% glucose). Continue to monitor the patient's blood pressure and if they become hypotensive, administer saline and raise the foot of the trolley.

There might be uncertainty as to whether or not this is a **TIA** or a stroke. However, even if it is a TIA, the risk of developing a stroke is greatest in the first 72 hours. Therefore, it is still vital to transfer to a specialist unit or a hospital with specialist services. Do not administer aspirin in the pre-hospital environment because while it is useful in the ischaemic stroke, it would make a haemorrhagic stroke more complicated.

A patient who has suffered a TIA and is properly investigated and treated has an 80% chance of not going on to having another episode or future stroke.

At the emergency department

On arrival at the emergency room, the crew hands over at the triage station to the specialist nurse. The important features to include are: time, course of symptoms and their evolution, position patient found in, likelihood of a fall/further complications or exclusion from mechanism of injury and any relevant collaborative history gathered that was not documented on the Patient Report Form (PRF). Make clear the main risk factors the patient is suffering from (and include positive negative findings, such as the patient was not incontinent at scene).

Key learning points

- Treatment is time dependent and faster treatment will improve the prognosis. Thrombolysis might or might not be required but early specialist care is still vital.
- A 12-lead ECG would be advisable en route to the hospital to check for AF. Intravenous access is not essential unless the patient requires specific intervention. Do not delay transport for tests, the priority is the patient reaching a specialist unit.

Summary

Stroke is a major health problem in the UK. Improving care for patients with stroke and transient ischaemic attack (TIA) is a key national priority, with a National Stroke Strategy published by the Department of Health in 2007, and guidelines published by the National Institute for Health and Clinical Excellence (NICE) in 2008.

Each year in England, approximately 110,000 people have a first or recurrent stroke and a further 20,000 people have a TIA.

Stroke accounted for over 56,000 deaths in England and Wales in 1999, which represents 11% of all deaths. Most people survive a first stroke, but often have significant morbidity. More than 900,000 people in England are living with the effects of stroke, with half of these being dependent on other people for help with everyday activities.

The majority (85%) of strokes are thrombotic (cerebral infarction) and 15% intracranial haemorrhage. Distinguishing between the two is not currently feasible in the pre-hospital setting. See Table 10.1 for the FAST test to assess a stroke.

Table 10.1 FAST

Face Weakness	Ask the patient to smile or show teeth. Look for NEW lack of symmetry.
Arm Weakness	Ask the patient to lift their arms together and hold for 5 seconds. Does one arm drift or fall down? The arm with motor weakness will drift downwards compared to the unaffected limb.
Speech	Ask the patient to repeat a phrase. Assess for slurring or difficulty with the words or sentence. These components make up the **FAST** (face, arms, speech test) assessment that should be carried out on **ALL** patients with suspected stroke/TIA. A deficit in any one of the three domains is sufficient for the patient to be identified as 'FAST positive'.
Time	It is essential to get this patient to a specialist unit as soon as possible.

REFERENCES

Department of Health (DoH) (2007) *National Stroke Strategy*. London: Department of Health.

National Institute for Health and Clinical Excellence (NICE) (2008) *Stroke: The Diagnosis and Initial Management of Acute Stroke and Transient Ischaemic Attack*. London: NICE.

FURTHER READING

Comprehensive, high-quality stroke information is available at:

NHS Evidence – Stroke   http://www.evidence.nhs.uk/specialistcollections.

NHS Stroke Improvement   http://www.improvement.nhs.

The Stroke Association   http://www.stroke.org.uk.

Case outline

Caroline Jones is a 64-year-old woman who was taken ill at her home after suffering with three days of colicky-like abdominal pain. During that period of time she had been feeling a degree of nausea and had vomited on a few occasions, including this morning.

When the paramedies arrive Caroline is lying on the settee, semi-recumbent, with her knees drawn up and a hot water bottle placed over her abdomen. A bowl is near her with evidence of yellow vomit which appears to be predominately bile.

The crew introduce themselves and, after conducting a visual primary survey, start asking what has happened while the driver/technician takes some baseline observations. Carol's lips are dry, she seems very fatigued and looks pale and unwell.

Baseline observations

Airway:	open and clear with a sour odour;
Breathing:	25 bpm regular;
Circulation:	110 bpm;
	BP is 125/80 mmHg;
Disability:	tired and fatigued but conscious;
	Glasgow Coma Scale = 15/15;
Blood glucose:	Normal at 5.9 mmol/L
Temperature:	37.4°C

She states that she has not moved her bowels for the last four days and her abdomen appears to be somewhat distended. She is anxious about her condition and states her pain score as 8 out of 10.

---

1   **What is your current differential diagnosis?**

A   **Constipation** can have a number of different causes and is an extremely common complaint. For some people, it isn't something they consider to be a symptom because it is part of their normal bowel habit. Therefore, one of your first questions about her bowel habit should be, 'how often is normal?'.

You should clarify what they mean by constipation. Is it simply that they haven't had a bowel movement/had no urge to go or that the stool is too hard and painful to pass?

The cause of her constipation could be one of the following:

- poor diet (lack of fibre);
- a result of medication (such as opioid pain relief, e.g. codeine);
- intestinal obstruction (e.g. bowel cancer);
- metabolic problems (e.g. hypothyroidism);
- lack of mobility.

Vomiting is a fairly non-specific symptom that may be related to her constipation or even to the pain she is in. We can't rule out food poisoning or even an overdose of pain relief that might have been self-medicated.

2 **How do we differentiate between these options and why?**

A Abdominal pain is one of the most common reasons why people might seek medical attention but it might be challenging to identify the specific cause of it due to the diversity of symptoms that the patient might present with.

Having considered the causes for her symptoms, the crew will also have to consider the fact that the lack of bowel movements might be due to the patient not having eaten anything. Ask the patient if they have ever had any pain like this before or if they have had any abdominal surgery. This might Indicate a recurrence of the previous problem, adhesions or post-operative infection.

Also the crew should obtain a detailed medication history – a patient taking multiple medications is at increased risk of damage to the liver, patients taking **NSAIDs** are at increased risk of gastric irritation/bleeding, another cause of pain but perhaps not the constipation. As discussed, however, opioid analgesia

> **Obstipation**
> Severe constipation caused by intestinal obstruction.

is associated with constipation. It is also worth considering whether the patient has a history of conditions such as **Crohn's disease** or **peptic ulcer** disease. Finally, in females it is important to consider pregnancy as acute abdominal pain in early pregnancy could be indicative of an ectopic pregnancy (Cole et al. 2006).

Given this patient's age and progression of symptoms, bowel obstruction seems the most likely diagnosis. To differentiate between a partial and complete obstruction depends on the patient's ability to pass gas. If they are able to, it is likely to be a partial obstruction due to constipation or possibly due to a growth (consider cancer) blocking the passage of faeces. If she is unable to pass any wind (or hasn't in the time she has also been constipated) suspect a complete obstruction. This could be due to twisting of the bowel, which is often as a result of adhesions or part of the bowel becoming displaced into a **hernia**. All of these options are a possibility in this patient and will require further investigations such as an abdominal X-ray to narrow down the cause.

> Adhesions are areas of post-surgical internal scar tissue, which could grow across the bowel causing twisting and blockage of the lumen.

3 **What is the pathophysiology behind Caroline's main symptoms?**

A See Table 11.1 for a list of possible causes of Caroline's symptoms.

Table 11.1 Pathophysiology behind Caroline's symptoms

Caroline's symptoms	Pathophysiology
Colicky abdominal pain	Generally occurs in the case of small bowel obstruction. Pain is often felt around the umbilical or epigastric areas of the abdomen. This occurs because of the natural peristaltic action of the gut. However if the large bowel was obstructed, it is more likely that the middle and lower abdomen will be affected with a gradual onset, cramp-like pain (Hughes 2005).
Nausea and vomiting	Due to the constipation, increased secretions from the bowel wall with no movement of fluid in to the intestinal lumen leads to fluid and electrolyte accumulation in the gut lumen. Fluid will therefore be passed back or backflow to the stomach, causing vomiting (Mattson Porth 2007). If the obstruction is high, the tendency for vomiting is particularly raised, and usually causes more severe vomiting (Baines 1998). Higher fluid levels are associated with the small bowel as the majority of fluid is absorbed after it passes through the **ileo-caecal valve** and vomiting occurs earlier with small bowel obstruction than large bowel (Hughes 2005).
No bowel movement	Small bowel obstruction may be due to hernias, adhesions, tumours or Crohn's disease. Large bowel obstructions are normally due to carcinoma or diverticulitis.
Tachycardia	Tachycardia can be linked to the compensatory mechanism associated with hypovolaemia.
Tachypnoea	The respiratory rate is increased as the heart and lungs work together to oxygenate the small volume of circulating blood. Increased respiratory rate is an early indicator of deterioration in the acutely unwell patient.
Distended abdomen	Due to the obstruction, fluids accumulate in the area. If untreated, the distension resulting from bowel obstruction tends to perpetuate itself by causing atony of the bowel and can lead to further distension. Distension will also be further aggravated by the accumulation of gases, the majority of which will be derived from swallowed air. Increased pressure in the intestine might compromise mucosal blood flow and ultimately may result in strangulation or interruption of blood flow to the bowel. This can cause necrosis, gangrenous changes and ultimately, perforation of the bowel (Mattson Porth 2007).

4   **What might be the initial management of Caroline?**

A   Initial management of intestinal obstruction is by fluid and electrolyte resuscitation and the use of a **naso-gastric (NG) tube** for aspiration and decompression of the bowel.

An increase in temperature, pulse rate, pain levels or white cell count will require further investigation as this could indicate a further deterioration in the patient's condition due to perforation of the bowel and risk of **sepsis** and **peritonitis**.

On assessment Caroline indicates her pain is at level 8 on a 0–10 pain tool.

5   **What type of pain relief should administer?**

A   As the pain is described as being quite severe in nature, the drug of choice is likely to be opioid analgesics as lower-grade analgesia such as entonox is not going to be helpful. It has been noted however that some doctors can be reluctant to use analgesia in case it masks clinical findings and therefore delays diagnosis. However, a Cochrane review evaluated clinical trials comparing administration of opioid analgesia to no analgesia in patients with acute abdominal pain (Manterola et al. 2007). The authors concluded that opioid analgesics were helpful in terms of patient comfort and did not mask clinical findings or delay prognosis. One of the side effects of these drugs is, however, constipation!

6   **How would you manage this patient's nausea and vomiting?**

A   **Metoclopramide** is commonly used in surgical settings and indeed in pre-hospital care for the management of nausea and vomiting. However, it is suggested that this drug might be contraindicated in the case of bowel obstruction due to its mode of action. Metoclopramide acts as a **prokinetic**, which stimulates gastric emptying. It will therefore further distend the bowel, as the stomach contents will pass into an area of the gut where there is no possible outlet. **Cyclizine**, however, acts on the chemoreceptor trigger zone and/or vomiting centre to block the neurotransmitters and therefore should not further compound the problem of distension (Hughes 2005).

Following initial investigations, Caroline Jones is admitted to a surgical ward. Initial investigations (in this case, abdominal X-ray) indicate that she has a small bowel obstruction.

Her vital signs are now:

Airway:	open and clear with a sour odour;
Breathing:	26 bpm regular;
Circulation:	125 bpm;
	BP is 105/60 mmHg;
Disability:	tired and fatigued but conscious;
	Glasgow Coma Scale = 15/15;
Blood glucose:	normal at 5.9 mmol/L;
Temperature:	38.5°C

Her **WCC** is raised at 16 (normal range 4–10).
The **arterial blood gas** (ABG) also indicates a metabolic acidosis.

7   **Explain why these observations/blood results could be abnormal in relation to the underlying pathophysiology.**

A   • **Temp 38.5°C** – the increased pressure in the intestine tends to compromise mucosal blood flow, which could lead to necrosis and movement of fluids into the **luminal fields**. This promotes rapid growth of bacteria in the obstructed bowel. **Anaerobes** grow rapidly in this favourable environment. If perforation does occur, it can rapidly lead to sepsis.

- **Pulse** – tachycardia can be linked to the compensatory mechanism associated with hypo-volaemia (indicated by the low blood pressure) as the heart attempts to circulate the lower blood volume.
- **RR** – increased to compensate for the hypovolaemia and also as a result of the pain. It is also worth noting, if distension is severe enough, it could push against the diaphragm and decrease lung volume.
- **WCC** – a raised WCC can be an indicator of infection. In this case it suggests perforation or sepsis as bowel contents empty into the peritoneal cavity.

Key learning points

- Constipation can be a surgical emergency, so rapid transfer for more investigations is required.
- Acute abdominal problems can run the risk of peritonitis due to a perforated bowel. Check regularly for signs of deterioration and sepsis.
- Have a good understanding of what the patient means by their symptoms (what might seem like constipation or diarrhoea to some might simply be a natural change in bowel habit rather than anything sinister).

REFERENCES

Baines, M.J. (1998) Nausea and vomiting. In: Fallon, M. and O'Neill, B. eds.: *ABC of Palliative Care*. London: BMJ Books, 1998: pp 16–18.

Cole, E., Lynch, A. and Cugnoni, H. (2006) Assessment of the patient with acute abdominal pain. *Nursing Standard* 20: 67–75.

Hughes, E. (2005) Caring for the patient with an intestinal obstruction. *Nursing Standard* 19: 56–64.

Manterola, C., Astudillo, P., Losada, H., Pineda, V., Sanhueza, A. and Vial, M. (2007) Analgesia in patients with acute abdominal pain. *Cochrane Database of Systematic Reviews* 3. Available at: http://www.cochrane.org/reviews.

Mattson Porth, C. (2007) *Essentials of Pathophysiology: Concepts of Altered Health States*. Philadelphia: Lippincott Williams and Wilkins.

CASE STUDY 12
Cut and run

Case outline

The funfair had arrived for the bank holiday weekend and the ambulance crew had been placed on active standby next to the common in preparation for any calls on the showground that might arise.

The call was to 'a fight by the dodgems'. Upon arrival, the crowds parted to reveal a young guy on the floor with dark red fluid covering one side of his pale tee-shirt.

The space was sufficient to see the worried and concerned faces of the bystanders and the ambulance crew was aware that the attacker might still be next to them in the crowd. Potential danger remained as they spoke to the patient, who was around 16 years of age, and his eyes tracked them in his own fear and obvious pain as his red hands grabbed his side.

Brief introductions were responded to with nods and a name, Shane. His breathing appeared to be in gasps and so although the crew were 'happy' with his airway at this stage, they quickly snipped up his tee-shirt to get a better look behind the red mess. A 2.5 cm-long wound of uncertain depth was on his chest. The attendant had already been ripping open a dressing and that was handed to the paramedic who placed it on the open wound with a reasonable amount of direct pressure. The blood loss was no more than around 500 ml externally, so although serious, external catastrophic haemorrhage was not the current issue.

1 **Besides the stab wound what else should the crew consider?**

A
- Secondary stab wounds.
- Kicks or punches to the body and the head.
- Has he been unconscious (very important, even if he is currently conscious)?
- Has he taken alcohol or drugs this evening?
- Is the weapon on the ground to see the size of the blade? (Useful information for hospital doctors in estimating extent of damage to internal organs.)

Initial observations and clinical findings were being assembled to give the crew a baseline and a secondary survey was under way with a quick neck-to-knees survey. Nothing obvious was found on the body and the story from his girlfriend matched with what was a robbery for a new fancy phone and a sharp pain in his side as the single knife wound was inflicted. The two thieves had disappeared and left the young man and his girlfriend screaming out.

Baseline observations

Danger: diminished (police arrived during the end of the primary survey);
Response: alert and a GCS of 15;
Airway: clear and he continued to be able to communicate to the crew;
Breathing: raised to 20 breaths per minute (but within normal boundaries);
Circulation: rapid, weak pulse at 140 bpm (pain, anxiety, and blood loss);
Disability: full movement, conscious prior to arrival, eyes PEARRL (size 4);
Exposure: showed single clean wound on right-hand side between rib 5 and 6;
                     weapon removed by attacker, and not found by the police in the imme-
                     diate area;
BP: 100/76 mmHg;
BM: 6.4 mmol/L;
Temperature: 36.8°C.

The paramedic decided to replace the dry dressings now soaked with blood with a new proprietary chest seal (**Asherman seal**) that allows air to escape out and stops any more being drawn in, on inspiration.

2   **What features would you expect to find on further examination of the chest?**

A   • Percussion of the chest might be hyperresonant (higher pitched) on the right side.
        • Auscultation (by stethoscope) might reveal clear breath sounds on left side but diminished on right side. There might be some crackles due to air being within the pleural space.

3   **What other chest wall signs can you look for?**

A   • Reduced chest wall movement of the affected side which might also be hyperexpanded (due to increased air going in, that cannot escape).
        • Mediastinal shift away from the affected side as the rising pressure of air entering the cavity pushes on the healthy lung.

4   **Why use an Asherman seal?**

A   The purpose is to reduce what appears to be a pneumothorax from tensioning. This dressing can also be used to stabilize a cannula used to decompress a pneumothorax (Allison et al. 2002). You could also use a dressing larger than the wound itself and secure on three sides to allow release of pressure but preventing more air entering the wound.

5   **How would you be able to tell the difference if a pneumothorax degraded to a tension pneumothorax?**

A   A pneumothorax is a collection of air in the pleural cavity of the chest between the lung and the chest wall. An opening in the chest wall creating this space will cause air to be pulled into the chest cavity by negative pressure and collapse the lung on the affected side. A pneumothorax can lead to hypoxia, an increasing respiratory rate and falling blood pressure due to compression of the heart and great vessels; this situation is termed tension pneumothorax. Therefore, you must keep monitoring the patient's obs. In a larger pneumothorax or tension pneumothorax, the air could be aspirated with a syringe/cannula (pre-hospital) or a one-way chest tube could be inserted to allow the air to escape (normally at hospital). However, the size of the pneumothorax doesn't bear any relationship to the severity of the symptoms experienced so treatment will depend on the condition of the patient.

The injury incurred in this patient is termed traumatic pneumothorax as it is from a stab wound. The incidence of a tension pneumothorax in the pre-hospital setting is around 5.4% (Coats et al. 1995).

A stab wound to the chest would automatically place this patient into a time-critical category as the internal damage and continued bleeding cannot be assessed in the field with any accuracy. The blood pressure is low but a second set of observations shows that Shane is not out of the woods yet.

6 **What other serious injuries might you be concerned about with a stab wound involving the chest wall?**

A Other than a pneumothorax, a haemothorax must be considered. This is when blood is trapped in the pleural cavity and is more likely in a stab wound where damage to the greater blood vessels has occurred. A pneumohaemothorax is when both blood and air are trapped (also a possibility in this case). Fluid pooling in the lungs can be a major cause of hypovolaemia (and resulting hypotension) in these cases.

7 **How would you treat this patient at the scene?**

A Shane would be immediately made ready for transfer to the nearest major trauma unit. The local helicopter with flight medics might be off line at night so there should be no delay in transfer to hospital by ground ambulance. Shane should be loaded on to the ambulance, lying semi-recumbent and marginally inclined to the injured side to aid any drainage.

A precautionary cannula is inserted in the anticubital fossa (ACF) but fluid challenges are not called for while his systolic blood pressure remains above 100. His signs and symptoms remain stable, suggesting no tension pneumothorax. However, if his obs did begin to change, it would be difficult to know if this was due to the pneumothorax created by the injury or to internal and unseen blood loss. To increase his blood pressure artificially may well increase his blood loss and the useful blood cells carrying his oxygen. Therefore, no release of the pneumothorax is needed at this stage and no fluids required, although placing a large bore cannula in each arm might be useful if fluids are suddenly indicated either on the way to hospital or on arrival at hospital. His oxygen saturation is maintained with oxygen via a NRB (non-rebreather) mask and he is placed in a comfortable position on his affected side. You would also want to provide the patient with analgesia as he is in serious pain from his injury.

As the crew began to move Shane into the ambulance, his condition suddenly worsened, his tachycardia increased and his demeanour became very quiet. The lead paramedic tries to rouse him but cannot get him to respond to verbal cues. His obs were taken again:

- airway remains patent;
- breathing is shallow and laboured with reduced chest wall movements;
- respiratory rate of 28 bpm is high and might show some early shock and compensatory mechanism kicking in for hypoxia;
- circulation is up with a heart rate of 130 bpm;
- blood pressure of 88/54 mmHg is slightly lower than is desirable.

8 **How would your management now change?**

A The change in his baseline observations suggests that he is either losing blood internally or his pneumothorax has worsened. The fact that his breathing is more labored and that his chest wall movements have reduced suggests it is due to the worsening pneumothorax and this will need to be treated immediately.

Start by maintaining the airway with a jaw thrust and continue high-flow oxygen via a non-rebreather (NRB) mask. Be prepared to place an airway if his breathing continues to deteriorate. Emergency needle decompression of the pneumothorax via needle thoracostomy is now vital. Place a large bore (14–16 G) intravenous cannula into the second rib space in the mid-clavicular line. Cannulae are unstable, prone to kinking, displacement or blockage and so should be rapidly replaced with a chest drain on arrival at hospital.

Support his circulation by giving IV fluids (into the already placed cannula) and move the patient into the supine (or trendelenburg) position to maintain blood flow to vital organs.

Therefore, either at handover or in advance of arrival, inform the emergency department that a needle thoracostomy has occurred so that they can prepare for a chest drain, if required. It also indicates the severity of the patient's condition, enabling the hospital team to be better prepared for the patient's arrival.

Shane will now need immediate transfer to the nearest major trauma centre by the fastest route available. A pre-alert call for this patient is vital.

Key learning points

- In violent trauma, such as this, be aware of ongoing danger and the risks you face going in to treat the patient. Request police presence if you become concerned at any point.
- Patients can deteriorate rapidly with chest wall injuries due to internal blood loss and damage to vital organs. Monitor vital signs closely and transfer to a trauma unit for optimum outcome for the patient.
- A tension pneumothorax can cause hypoxia, tachypnoea and hypotension due to compression of the heart and great vessels.

REFERENCES

Allison, K., Porter, K.M. and Mason, A.M. (2002) Use of the Asherman chest seal as a stabilisation device for needle thoracostomy. *Emergency Medicine Journal* 19: 590–91.

Coats, T.J., Wilson, A.W. and Xeropotamous, N. (1995) Pre-hospital management of patients with severe thoracic injury. *Injury* 2: 581–5.

FURTHER READING

Driscoll, P., Skinner, D. and Earlam, R. (eds) (2007) *ABC of Major Trauma*. London: BMJ Books.

Knowing your limits

Case outline

Excess alcohol consumption in all age groups, especially the teenager population, has become an increasingly common problem. Alcohol-related calls continue to take up a significant volume of ambulance responses.

Gillian Oakdean lives on her own and consumes her time and her pension with regular trips to the Leicester Arms round the corner and also the off-licence at the corner of her street. She has always been a sociable person and knows a large number of the local neighbours as she has lived in the same road for over 43 of her 67 years. Today a friend called in to see how she was doing and was so concerned on her findings that she immediately called an ambulance.

Responding to an adult female vomiting blood is a routine call, yet unusual at 9 in the morning. The crew donned gloves as they entered the front door and were met with quite a scene. The smell of alcohol and vomit in the dimly lit room with the curtains drawn was quite overpowering. The biggest danger here is to assume that this is just another drunk who needs to sleep it off and the desire to conduct a cursory examination and get out with or without the patient has to be overcome.

A couple of table lamps revealed a couple of full waste paper bins with an assortment of wine bottles and cans. Some bottles lay strewn on the floor, causing stained puddles on the carpet. Cigarette ash poured over the ashtray, with rubbish covering every surface.

Initial baseline observations

Safety:	caution throughout but initially low risk;
Airway:	clear, although her breath was quite difficult to be close to;
Breathing:	18 breaths per minute;
Circulation:	weak and thready radial pulse was 110 bpm and the deeply sunken and gaunt eyes were in keeping with her overly thin frame;
Disability:	GCS of around 15 as Gillian was close to sober, having been sick much of the night and not having had any alcohol for the past eight hours;
General appearance:	Gillian was considerably unkempt and her hair was matted to her head in a combination of sweat and dirt;
BP:	120/85 mmHg;
BM:	5.4 mmol/L;
Temperature:	36.5°C.

On examination, the vomit in one of the bowls was predominantly bile, with a fair amount of red blood streaked through it. Her tender abdomen was causing the patient to lean over as she sat on the edge of the chair. Her skin had a definite yellowish, tawny colour with the yellow colour also being seen in the conjunctiva of her eyes suggestive of jaundice.

> **Cirrhosis** is derived from the Greek word κιρρός [*kirrós*] which means yellowish, describing the orange-yellow colour of the skin seen in chronic liver disease.

After peeling off the sleeve of her matted sweater a blood pressure was obtained at 164/98 mmHg and her temperature was slightly lowered at 36.5°C. Her pallor and cracked lips suggested she was dehydrated. Her fingers showed some signs of **clubbing** (the angle between the nail and proximal nail fold is more than 180 degrees). The palms of her hands looked slightly red (palmar erythema) and her chest was covered in small, red dots

> **Spider naevi** are caused by vascular changes where a central arteriole has multiple small vessels branching away from the centre, seen on the surface of the skin as a red, spider-like lesion.

that were not rash-like but more in keeping with the effect known as **spider naevi**.

With some difficulty, her abdomen was examined (**IAPP**) where the liver was nodular but was not enlarged.

---

1   **What is the differential diagnosis of these signs?**

A
- Jaundice can have multiple causes (normally divided into pre-hepatic, hepatic and post-hepatic) and is not the only sign shown by this patient. Jaundice alongside nodular liver changes would make you concerned about liver **cirrhosis**.
- Liver cirrhosis causes include high alcohol intake (suspected in this patient given the findings in her home), chronic viral hepatitis (e.g. hepatitis C), metabolic or inherited disorders (such as haemochromatosis) and as a side effect of drugs.

The crew have so far been unable to gather enough information to distinguish between these possibilities. One of the first questions you would need to ask is if the patient has ever experienced anything like this before or does she have any known problems with her liver? An inherited disorder might already be known by the patient but can still be an unknown entity. Take a full alcohol and drug history. Intravenous drug use can lead to the transmission of hepatitis as can unprotected sex. These are questions you might not wish to ask in the pre-hospital setting but are worth considering.

Other than illicit drugs, also ask about medication and over-the-counter (including herbal) remedies. Many prescription drugs require constant liver monitoring due to possible liver damage in the same way that some seemingly safe and natural herbal remedies can lead to extensive liver disease.

Although there is no single sign that the condition is **pathognomonic**, the most likely cause in this patient is going to be alcoholic liver disease. The other signs (spider naevi, **palmar erythema**, jaundice) and symptoms (nausea, vomiting, bleeding) she is experiencing are all in keeping with cirrhotic liver disease due to chronic alcohol abuse.

An important fact to remember here is that alcoholic liver disease doesn't just occur in alcoholics; genetics can make some people very sensitive to the effects of alcohol due to an inability to metabolize alcohol at the normal rate.

Gillian was drinking around two to three bottles of wine a day (much more than the recommended weekly consumption of 14 units for a female and daily consumption of 2–3 units). There was some distention of her abdomen, remarkable on her slight frame, most likely to be due to **ascites** (fluid retention in the abdominal cavity). Gillian's long-term outcome along with her advanced liver cirrhosis is not good and it might not be possible to reverse the process of damage without a liver transplant. She does not have

> **Units of alcohol**
> 1 unit = 8 mg (or 10 ml) of pure alcohol. While this varies with each type of alcoholic drink, a general guide is half a pint of 3.5% beer/lager or cider, a 125 ml glass of 9% wine or a 25 ml measure of 40% spirits.

any known liver disease or viral hepatitis and is not currently taking any medication or herbal remedies. She is unable to recall information when asked and appears confused when questioned about previous medical conditions saying that she can't remember.

2 **What other physical problems are you concerned about in chronic alcohol abuse?**

A (a) **Wernicke's encephalopathy** can be associated with alcohol use and is associated with **thiamine (vitamin B12)** deficiency. Symptoms to look for include abnormal eye movements (e.g. **nystagmus**), **ataxia** with a wide, unstable gait and short-term memory loss.

(b) Chronic alcoholics can also suffer with gastritis, **splenomegaly** and splenic rupture (a surgical emergency). Oesophageal **varices** are also a common feature due to dilated veins as a result of portal hypertension (another consequence of liver cirrhosis), leading to bleeding on vomiting.

(c) Patients who are withdrawing from alcohol can suffer with delirium tremens or alcohol-withdrawal seizures. Delirium tremens is an acute neurological and mental change in response to alcohol withdrawal. It can be confused with psychosis due to perceptual abnormalities and visual and tactile hallucinations, classically involving insects. Both require immediate hospital referral for assessment and treatment.

3 **How does high alcohol consumption lead to liver cirrhosis?**

A The metabolism of alcohol occurs in the liver, producing toxins that require excretion. This process also causes an increase in inflammatory cytokines with the inflammation causing damage to hepatocytes (cells making up the liver) over repeated exposure. Because the liver is able to regenerate, it replaces damaged hepatocytes with scar tissue (fibrosis) which causes the nodules to form on the surface of the liver.

The fibrous changes to the liver make the normal blood flow through the liver more difficult and affect the blood supply to the organ which is what causes portal hypertension.

4   **Why do people with liver disease also have bleeding problems?**

A   The liver is where all clotting factors are produced (except F VIII). All factors are involved in the coagulation cascade: the conversion of each factor into the next that leads to the formation of a fibrin clot and cessation of bleeding from a wound. Disruption of the function of the liver (in both acute and chronic disease) causes production of these factors to be diminished. This risks prolonged bleeding from a wound and associated acute hypotension and hypovolaemic shock.

The liver also produces bile salts which are involved in the absorption of vitamin K in the GI system. Vitamin K is an important co-enzyme in the production of clotting factors and so its absence will also reduce the clotting ability of the patient.

5   **Why is alcohol consumption such a problem to society?**

A   Don't always believe the stereotypes; yes young people tend to binge drink and drink heavily but older people tend to drink more regularly. Both are damaging to the liver. NHS (2007) statistics show that while guidance is in place, 24% of men and 13% of women report drinking on average more than the recommended units per week. The same report shows that in 2005, 6570 people in England and in Wales died from causes directly related to alcohol consumption (two-thirds of these patients died from alcoholic liver disease), costing the NHS £1.4 and £1.7 billion per year. The recommended units of alcohol are in place to help people drink within what is considered a 'healthy' limit to reduce the likelihood of developing the complications of excess alcohol consumption.

Key learning points

- Liver disease requires extensive investigation in the hospital setting and accurate diagnosis is rarely possible in the pre-hospital setting.
- Complications of chronic liver disease can be serious and require emergency treatment. It is important to be aware of these when assessing these patients.

REFERENCE

NHS (2007) National Statistics, The Statistics on Alcohol: England. The Information Centre. Available [online] at http://www.ic.nhs.uk/pubs/alcohol07

FURTHER READING

NICE (2010) *Alcohol-use Disorders: Preventing the Development of Hazardous and Harmful Drinking*. London: NICE.

Slips, trips and falls

Case outline

'Fall, query assist', was on the mobile data terminal (MDT) as the crew weaved slightly cautiously along the side roads at 3 am in response to a call. There was no one waving them down on arrival, but a light was on in the hall and the door ajar.

The crew selected a response pack (including an AED) plus some oxygen therapy equipment in a barrel bag. The crew double-checked the number on the house wall and eased open the door, calling out to the potential patient as they entered.

On the ground floor in the hall reclined a male in his late 50s who greeted them with a smile and a raised hand that had been holding his leg. 'Hi, sorry to call you out, but I've slipped and fallen on the bath mat when I got up for a leak, just need a hand up'. When asked what happened, the patient replied that he slipped on the bath mat and was in a lot of pain but has managed to drag himself into the hallway towards the phone.

On further questioning, Lorenz, a 55-year-old construction worker, described his anxiety about the pain in his hip and at the top of his right leg, telling the crew he cannot be off work. He describes the pain as the worst he has ever had and that he was unable to stand up (he attempted to stand to reach for the phone). On observation, the leg appears abnormally rotated and is being held very still as the patient flinched in pain if moved. He described no loss of consciousness and had been on the floor for around 20 minutes.

Concerned that he might have sustained a fracture, the crew want to ensure his baseline observations are stable before attempting to transfer him anywhere.

Baseline observations

Response:	alert and a GCS of 15;
Airway:	clear, the patient is talking coherently to the crew;
Breathing:	raised to 25 breaths per minute (due to the pain and anxiety);
Circulation:	slightly raised at 110 bpm (pain and anxiety);
Disability:	patient is conscious but currently immobile;
Exposure:	lying in his boxers and a tee-shirt with no obvious skin wounds; clothing would need to be removed to fully assess this but is likely to be done at the emergency room;
BP:	130/85 mmHg;
BM:	6.4 mmol/L;
Temperature:	36.8°C.

1   **What type of fracture are you concerned about?**

A   Pain in this region and with the mode of injury would be most likely to be caused by a fracture in the neck or the shaft of the femur. Also consider if there has been any involvement of the pelvis. A pelvic fracture is also associated with severe blood loss so you would monitor blood pressure and heart rate very closely.

> The **femur** is the longest bone and is one of the two strongest bones in the body (the other being the temporal bone). The average adult male femur is 48 cm (18.9 in.) in length and 2.34 cm (0.92 in.) in diameter and can support up to 30 times the weight of an adult.

2   **Why are fractured femurs so important?**

A   Fractures in this region in young people are associated with high-impact trauma (e.g. a road traffic collision) or a fall from a great height. In the elderly, these fractures are common after a simple trip due to osteoporotic changes in their bones, making them more fragile. The femur is a very strong bone so for a fracture to occur a large force has to be applied unless the bone is already damaged and weakened. Given the mode of injury, this is a fairly low-impact event. This patient is also relatively young for a fracture to be due to **osteoporosis** and while this could still be the case, other pathology must be considered as the underlying cause.

Bones can be weakened by a tumour in the area that has fractured or due to infection. These conditions are termed pathologic femur fractures. Therefore, ask the patient if they have any known conditions that caused the fracture and can be flagged up at arrival to hospital. It is, however, unlikely that this will be known and can actually lead to the presentation of a sinister disease process that the patient is unaware of.

3   **How would you manage this patient for transfer?**

A   You would want to immobilize a mid-shaft fracture with a traction splint applied to the patient in a recumbent position. The fracture will then be reduced in hospital (under local or general anaesthetic) and then held via a back-slab or plaster. A fracture in the femur or hip is more likely to require surgical intervention to hold it in place. This might be via an intramedullary pin (pin going into the middle of the bone to hold the two parts together), plate and screws, wires and traction or prosthesis (joint replacement).

The patient is likely to be in a lot of pain so analgesia (e.g. morphine) should be considered. Reducing and holding the fracture in hospital will also help ease the level of pain but this is something you cannot do in the pre-hospital setting as imaging and further assessment will be required.

4   **Why are some patients more likely to fracture bones in low impact injuries?**

A   Elderly patients have degenerative change to their bones and joints, making them weaker and more prone to serious injury with only a small amount of impact. Fractured neck of femur is the most likely problem here and certain types of fracture in this region of the hip joint will require a hip replacement.

> **Who gets fractures?**
> The Department of Health tells us the number of hip fractures are rising, reflecting the ageing population. The mean age of those with a hip fracture is 75 years but the risk rises with increasing age. Hip fracture is considerably more common in elderly women than men (Fairbank et al. 1999)

This type of injury carries a high mortality rate in the elderly. The elderly can also be very isolated and falls at home, where they cannot get help quickly, can lead to dehydration and electrolyte imbalances that require correction in hospital before they can be operated on. Increased time between injury and treatment leads to poor prognosis and increased mortality. Factors that contribute to an increased risk of a fall in the elderly include a decline in vision, balance, sensory perception, strength and neuromuscular function.

5 **What should we be aware of related to a fractured neck of femur?**

A There are two types of fracture in the neck of femur: **intracapsular** and **extracapsular**. The neck of the femur has a limited blood supply and those that occur in the intracapsular region can lead to avascular necrosis as this fragile blood supply is disrupted. Treatment depends on age of the patient and how many hours since the fracture occurred. Commonly, and especially in the elderly, hip replacement is the best treatment but in younger patients, preserving the hip by realigning the joint is preferable. Early treatment is therefore vital as the longer the time between the fracture and treatment, the poorer the prognosis so it is important to establish when the fracture occurred.

6 **What causes osteoporosis?**

A Osteoporosis is the most common cause of bone weakening in older people. It is due to a reduction in bone minerals and the bone matrix with a significantly reduced bone mass. The effects are mostly seen in women after the menopause (due to hormonal changes leading to declining levels of oestrogen). Important risk factors for osteoporosis include increasing age, early menopause/late menarche (overall reduced oestrogen exposure), poor nutrition, reduced exercise, smoking and alcohol consumption.

Treatment and transport options

Full secondary survey (to rule out other potential injuries) in non-time critical patients is essential while selecting analgesia. Pain relief is a must as all large bone fractures are generally very painful. Dependent on mechanism of injury, ensure that primary care has supported the cervical vertebrae. Keep the patient warm as they have often been on a cool floor for some period of time before help arrived. A combination of blood loss, hypothermia and shock makes for a poor prognosis.

Traction splints work well on singular or bilateral mid-shaft of femurs but are generally either not applicable or unwise to use on neck of **femur**. There are a couple of new devices for securing hips but the older and more well established strap and support spring technique will still suffice in most cases.

Major trauma centre should be considered if available in your area. Give an appropriate alert call prior to arrival.

Key learning points

- Fracture occurrence is dependent on the type of injury as well as multiple patient factors.

- Assessing the risk factors for osteoporosis can help you identify when a fracture has occurred in an elderly patient.
- If the symptoms for a fractured femur seem to be more severe than you would expect for this mode of injury, be suspicious of underlying pathology.
- Know how to use your immobilization equipment, infrequently used but often forgotten.

REFERENCE

Fairbank, J., Goldacre, M., Mason, A., Wilkinson, E., Fletcher, J., Amess, M., Eastwood, A. and Cleary, R. (eds) (1999) *Health Outcome Indicators: Fractured Proximal Femur. Report of a working group to the Department of Health*. Oxford: National Centre for Health Outcomes Development.

Case outline

The crew received a call one morning to a home in a small village where a 14-year-old girl, Flora, had been complaining of a tummy ache for over 18 hours which had recently become worse, localizing on the right side.

Flora looked very pale and clammy, lying on the sofa on her side, clutching a pillow to her stomach. She had been to the toilet eight times overnight, and emptying the bowels or passing wind did not relieve the pain. There was no blood or mucus in the stool and she had now stopped going to the toilet altogether as she had had so little to eat or drink. She was unable to eat; she vomited when attempting a meal and then when she tried to drink water. The vomit was either clear or simply the colour of what she had eaten, producing no blood. It was now 20 hours since she had last eaten and 10 hours since she last had any water. The diarrhoea and vomiting have left her feeling weak and dehydrated. She appeared listless and exhausted.

Baseline observations

GCS:	13, there is a reduced response to questioning, at times she can appear confused;
Airway:	open and clear;
Breathing:	RR 22 bpm;
Circulation:	HR 110 bpm;
BP:	102/69 mmHg;
Blood glucose:	BM 4.5 mmol/L;
Temperature:	39.1°C.

1 How would you interpret these baseline observations given the history of the patient's symptoms?

A Flora's tachycardia and high respiratory rate are likely to be as a result of a combination of the pain and might also be influenced by the pathology behind it if there is inflammation due to infection. A high respiratory rate and heart rate would make you suspect infection, especially in the absence of pain. Her blood pressure is relatively normal but this should be monitored as a sudden drop would suggest septic shock and her level of potential dehydration

Glucose

In any patient who has a reduced conscious level it is vital that the blood or urine is checked for sugar level. The expression DEFG (Don't Ever Forget Glucose) is a very helpful prompt.

might be reflected in this as well. Blood glucose should be measured in all patients (**DEFG**) with altered conscious level (Flora is feeling listless and drowsy) but might also be slightly lower when a patient hasn't eaten and has been vomiting. Be aware that sepsis can also cause a glucose imbalance. It is, however, useful information to have to hand as an abnormal result should be presented on handover.

2 **What is important for you to establish from the history that will influence your management plan?**

A
- Level of dehydration: is she in hypovolaemic shock?
- Take a second blood pressure. Comparative is better than singular readings.
- Re-check GCS conscious state, gain from the history an estimate of her fluid balance from intake and losses.
- Any obvious internal or external blood loss?
- Any previous episodes or significant medical history?

If the patient is in shock, she will need rapid fluid challenge to restore fluid balance and emergency transfer to the nearest emergency department for further support. You would want to place a large-bore cannula for fluid resuscitation (en route or on arrival at hospital) and possibly take bloods (full blood count, U&Es and inflammatory markers, as per local protocols) to aid further investigation and diagnosis. The patient is likely to have more bloods taken at hospital, including group and save and a cross-match in order to prepare the patient should surgery be required.

On further examination, as part of the secondary survey, Flora tensed as the paramedic tried to touch her stomach; the area where she was in the most pain was in the right iliac fossa (Figure 15.1). She explained that the pain had originally been in no specific area and then moved down towards the right side and above the pelvis.

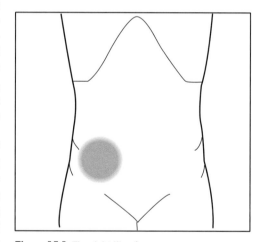

Figure 15.1 The right iliac fossa

---

3 **What is the differential diagnosis?**

A
- Inflammatory bowel disease (such as Crohn's or ulcerative colitis).
- Ectopic pregnancy.
- Gastroenteritis.

- Appendicitis.
- Ruptured ovarian cyst.

The best approach with the differential is to consider the anatomy of the area. Where the pain has localized to is where you will find the junction between the large and small bowel. Considering the pathology of the small bowel you would be concerned about inflammatory bowel disease, gastroenteritis or small bowel obstruction. In the large bowel, think about large bowel obstruction (**volvulus**, intussusception, cancer, constipation), inflammatory bowel disease, caecal mass blocking ileo-caecal valve, acute appendicitis and referred pain due to inflammation in the peritoneal cavity. In females, ovarian pathology can produce pain in this area as well so consider a ruptured ovarian cyst or ectopic pregnancy or endometriosis (although this is unlikely to produce such an acute event). In women of reproductive age, acute pain in this region is often considered to be an ectopic pregnancy until proven otherwise.

More specific paediatric problems to consider in this patient and those of younger age is bowel obstruction (although they are unlikely to have diarrhoea as well); incarcerated hernia, intussusception of bowel or **malrotated** bowel in young children.

This patient is of paediatric age but is likely to also present with some adult problems, especially considering that she is of child-bearing age and classically appendicitis and ectopic pregnancies have the same history, so on arrival to hospital a pregnancy test will always be carried out to exclude this as a cause of her symptoms. Once ectopic pregnancy is excluded, it is most likely that this patient would have appendicitis.

4 **Given the possible diagnosis, what changes in the patient's status would you need to monitor for?**

A Level of consciousness and dehydration. If there is an acute abdominal problem (e.g. acute appendicitis) you are most worried about the situation becoming worse such as the patient entering into septic shock. If the appendix is not removed, the area will become more inflamed and necrosis of the tissue begins. This weakens the tissue and makes perforation more likely. As you do not know the level of necrosis or severity of the stage of disease, it is important to transfer them to the nearest emergency department where they are likely to receive basic resuscitation in terms of fluids, oxygen and pain relief to stabilize their state prior to surgical review. The appendix will either be surgically removed or the patient will be conservatively treated with antibiotics and monitored to avoid surgery if this is deemed unnecessary.

5 **Why does the pain begin in the umbilicus before localizing to the right iliac fossa?**

A This works on the basis of referred pain. This is due to the initial embryological origins of organs and tissues affecting the nervous system. The appendix originates from the mid-gut structures in the development of the intestines. The initial pain from the organ is therefore referred straight from the dermatome of T10 and so is felt by the patient as a diffuse colicky pain (usually around the umbilicus). As the organ and surrounding peritoneum becomes more inflamed, the pain is then able to localize via a different nervous system and overrides the previous signals from T10 so the pain now feels like a constant pain in the right iliac fossa.

6 **What hospital investigations might be performed to confirm a diagnosis?**

A To rule out ectopic pregnancy, a pregnancy test would need to be performed. You would also want a full blood count and inflammatory markers. In acute appendicitis you would expect to see a raised white cell count, known as a leucocytosis (usually, high levels of **neutrophils** will be found). Due to the inflammation, a raised inflammatory marker called CRP (**C-reactive protein**) might be found to be raised as well.

Imaging (often ultrasound) will show an enlarged appendix and confirm a diagnosis of appendicitis.

As you are unable to complete investigations in the pre-hospital setting, your major focus in the management of a potential appendicitis case is to take a relevant history to assist hospital staff in excluding other causes for the abdominal pain. You would also want to complete all basic examinations to ensure the patient is stable when handing over and to be monitoring for a decline in the patients basic observations.

Appendicitis

There were nearly 40,000 emergency admissions between 2009 and 2010 due to appendicitis, making it a fairly common diagnosis in cases of abdominal pain.

Key learning points

- All acute pain in the right iliac fossa in women of child-bearing age should have ectopic pregnancy as the major diagnosis until proven otherwise by pregnancy testing.
- Not all cases of appendicitis require surgery but they are still an emergency, therefore rapid transfer is required. Dehydration and sepsis are two major causes for concern in patients with acute abdominal pain.
- Teenage patients should have both paediatric and adult causes for symptoms considered.

Case outline

The last call for the day arrives at 10.45 pm. The shift is nearly over but this call will take the crew past their 11:00 pm finish. They are called to a young woman in a kitchen fire. The paramedics naturally question how serious it could be. Hot drink spilt, a chip pan fire, scald from a gas flame on the cooker? They begin to think about what kit will be needed for the call, which is likely to involve burns and/or smoke inhalation.

Modern crews have access to a full burns kit, no longer relying on tap water and clean dry dressings. The range is quite varied and the crew don't get to use them often as burns are a relatively uncommon call (0.4%). Burns units are also few and far between so the decision whether to take to local ED or on to a specialist unit will be determined by severity of patient's condition, percentage of surface burned area and running time to the 'local centre'.

Pulling up outside the house, the paramedics see no Fire Service; does that mean the house is not on fire? The house appears calm with no one outside; this is a good sign as a house fire tends to attract a big crowd. In addition a rapid response car is turning into the same road on blues as the crew walk up the path to investigate.

A primary response kit will have a defibrillator, aspirator, dressings, simple airway adjuncts and a variety of water-soluble gelatine burn dressings. The oxygen barrel bag is essential, as burns patients tend to have burnt airways in severe cases due to breathing in very hot fumes. The bag contains all you need to support the breathing patient. Entonox is even better as it gives oxygen and some pain relief; however, it depends on the capability of the patient to draw in deep enough breaths as smoke inhalation and heat damage can cause the airways to swell and close up.

Danger

We don't wish to become patients ourselves, so don't rush in if not sure of the situation, and make sure the scene is dynamically safe. A knock on the door and a ring of the bell for good measure is met with an anxious woman (the patient's flatmate) who says 'this way, quick'.

Leaning over the sink in the kitchen is a young woman aged about 30 who has a wet tea towel over her back.

Response

The woman is alert and crying out in pain. Her back was severely burnt when the nightdress she was wearing caught fire from the gas stove as she turned around while making a hot drink for bed. The material caught light and melted on to the back and neck also causing her hair to briefly ignite. The scorched twisted blond hair is now frizzed up and shortened by about 18″ apart from a few strands at the sides and front. There is a large area, approximately 15–20%, of burnt flesh. The skin colour is predominately red with some white patches and a number of solid and burst blisters which are weeping across the dermis. Her front is not damaged by direct flame, although the kitchen has an acrid burnt smell that is very obvious and potent as soon as the crew walk in.

Primary survey is completed by the assisting paramedic with particular emphasis on the airway while the lead paramedic assesses the burnt skin.

Baseline observations

Response: good, at no time has the patient been unconscious;

Airway: clear and dry, unaffected by the burn, which was to the posterior of the patient. Few of the fumes were breathed in;

Breathing: steady at 18 bpm, slightly elevated as the patient is in pain and is anxious due to the trauma;

Circulation: raised at 110 bpm, but not unexpected due to the exposed burnt flesh and her pain response;

Disability: preferring to stand as she has good mobility;

Exposure: small fragments of the nightdress are in the wound and will need to be sorted at hospital. The percentage is agreed as 18% (her back);

Temperature: raised slightly at 37.4°C. A core temperature would be more useful at this stage, but not generally available in pre-hospital care;

BM: 6.0 mmol/L;

O$_2$ sats: 96% and is not requiring interventions at this stage.

1   **What is the first thing to consider?**

A   (a) Get her out and convey the lady rapidly to hospital?
(b) Stay and dress the wounds?
(c) Take a history and carry out a full secondary survey?

The key issue in this scenario is shock, so answers **b, a, c** are the best-ordered choice. However, don't stay long on scene even though her baseline figures indicate stability; **c** can occur en route to definitive care. The surface area that is damaged and exposed is allowing the hot skin to draw blood from the system to cool itself. The second critical area is to slow down or avoid overcooling which can lead to hypothermia and in itself more shock. Therefore, it is important to place a dressing but monitor the patient closely for signs of overcooling and hypothermia. Fluid is lost from burns injuries and patients often become dehydrated. Give IV 0.9% saline or Hartmann's for severe burns or when the transfer to hospital is going to be lengthy (more than one hour). However, cannulation should not be undertaken at the expense of rapid transfer to hospital. More accurate fluid calculations will be made in hospital based on the extent of the burns.

A calm approach is essential. The caller and her friend are looking for leadership and support in a terrible crisis. Lifting the tea towel away to quickly assess the area does two things: it allows the crew to see the surface area and depth of burn, although the second element is very difficult in these very early stages. The full effect of the burn will continue to deepen over the next few minutes if the heat is not adequately dissipated.

2   **What is your management approach?**

A   Change the now warm tea towel (wet dressing) for another cooler one, or swap the dressing for a proprietary burns dressing. A burns kit has been brought in with larger water-based dressings and a large dry sterile sheet. Some soft crepe bandage/dressings, lightly applied can also be used, to help secure the water-based dressings, but remember these are cool to the touch, not cold. As the dressings are cooling and given the loss of skin barrier which would normally help to retain heat, keep the patient warm by wrapping a blanket or clean clothing around her if necessary.

Other dressing options include using clingfilm as it maintains the wound appearance making further assessment on arrival to the burns unit much easier. However, clingfilm does not cool the burn and should only be considered when the pre-hospital treatment with water-based jell dressings is concluded. It also provides a protective barrier to the damaged skin. Avoid using flamazine dressings (silver sulphadiazine cream used to prevent infection) in immediate referrals as it makes assessment of the wound more difficult (Hettiaratchy and Papini 2004).

Give analgesia, ideally via intravenous route (giving an opioid) and give Entonox if required or if struggling to gain IV access. The main analgesia will come from the cooling dressing and should be the main priority. 'Cool, cover and convey' is the mantra of the day.

Put a Jell dressing in place and cover the exposed area by several spare centimetres. Pain relief is then administered while a dressing gown is wrapped around the patient's shoulders. She is not feeling cold, yet, but it is essential to prevent overcooling at this stage. The Jell dressing will draw heat for many minutes to allow the crew to package and get the patient out to the vehicle.

IV cannulation can be put off at this stage as the patient has peripherally shut down veins and in reality doesn't require large-volume fluids even though she has potential to fall into a shocked state. Fortunately the patient has not been smeared with cooking oil, grease, butter or even toothpaste; paramedics in previous cases of burns have witnessed all of these. The burn surgeons will soon need to see the wound and not have to clean off oil-based rubbish to get a good view.

The helpful rapid responder has been gathering a history from the flat mate of basics such as name, address, allergies, DOB, and has even gained background extras such as blood group and GP's name and address.

The patient asks to walk and the crew agrees this as there is no room to get a stretcher in the house passageway and the chair will be very painful to sit in with her back being pressed upon it.

In the vehicle the patient asks for the towelling dressing gown to be loosened to relieve any excess pressure on her back and they decide on the destination hospital. She sits on the trolley and supports herself in as comfortable a position as possible, taking in some Entonox to make her as comfortable as possible.

The patient is persuaded to receive a cannula in her left arm and she will soon receive 10 mg of morphine, which will help enormously on the 20-minute run to the burns centre in the next town. The crew decide not to change the Jell dressing as it has now maintained a reasonable air seal and has allowed natural cooling to draw the heat out with excessively damaging core temperature. Jell dressings have the advantage of normalizing temperature after 10–15 minutes and do not overcool, as long as the patient is secondary wrapped against wind chill factors.

3 **What are some other important types of burns?**

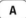
- Scalds (hot liquids).
- Contact burns (hot solid).
- Chemicals (acids or alkalis).
- Electrical burns (high and low voltage).
- Sunburn.

Treatment for scalds contact and sunburn are all very similar to this case study. Should there be burns of an entire limb or even the trunk of the patient, be cautious for restricted blood flow as the skin tightens under expansion. The hospital is able to perform an **escharotomy** to release and control the pressure.

4 **How would you manage chemical or electrical burn?**

A **Chemical burn**

Avoid constricting the area with tight dressings, instead irrigating the wound and using wet dressings only. However, if the burn is due to a powdered chemical, water would make it worse, so remove clothing, brush off chemical if possible and use dry dressings in these cases. Do not try and neutralize the causative chemical.

Electrical burn

Switch off power source or safely remove patient from source using non-conductive material (e.g. rubber or wood). Do not approach a patient connected to a high voltage source. Look for both entry and exit wounds, treat both areas.

> **Key learning points**
>
> - Remember not to overlook the primary survey in burns cases, however severe the injury may look.
> - Modern Jell dressings will help to cool the burn, halting further damage and provide a level of analgesia. However, like any cooling agents, monitor and protect from hypothermia.
> - Ideally place at least one cannula (in non-burnt skin) in order to allow fluid resuscitation, most likely to occur in hospital after calculation of fluid requirement but you may need to give fluids in severe burns or longer transfer times.

REFERENCES

Davis, S.C., Gil, J., Valdes, J., Claro, A., and Badiavas, E. (2010) *Second-degree burn wound study.* University of Miami.

Hettiaratchy, S. and Papini, R. (2004) Initial management of a major burn: I-overview. *BMJ* 328(7455): 1555–7.

Case outline

When an 8-year-old girl (Sadie) was taken ill in the schoolyard at morning break, a diligent playground monitor was able to alert the school office and put into action the school emergency health plan. The teacher on duty, who was first-aid trained, recognized the girl's serious difficulty in breathing and decided that being safe and calling an ambulance was the wisest move.

The crew arrived and drove into a now rapidly emptying schoolyard and pulled up by the front entrance, being cautious to drive at a moderate pace in the school grounds. The Deputy Head walked the crew along the corridor to the first aid room as the crew pulled the stretcher with them along with kit balanced on it.

Difficulty in breathing can be related to a number of causes both medical and traumatic. The crew naturally selected a portable oxygen bag along with the response bag containing the defibrillator. On arrival, the child was sat on the side of the first aid bed with her legs over the side. She appeared quite distressed and was struggling to breath. Her face was blotched and her eyes rolled around the room.

Baseline observations

Response: Sadie was responding to verbal stimulus and tracking the crew with her eyes but was unable to speak;

Airway: her airway appeared to be fine but with a clear whistling sound as though there might be a restriction;

Breathing: the respiratory rate was raised above normal at 30 breaths per minute;

Circulation: pulse is tachycardic at around 140 bpm at her radius. She is also hypotensive with a blood pressure of 95/65 mmHg;

Disability: her pupils appeared to be around size 4 at first glance;

Temperature: 36.9°C, considered close to normal;

BM: 7.5 mmol/L;

SpO$_2$ sats: she is mildly hypoxic at 94% but currently able to compensate with the rapid breathing rate.

Sadie's lips were relatively swollen and slightly blue and her face appeared pale. There were also signs of a red rash on her neck and chest. Her heart rate is regular and both heart sounds were heard, with no additional sounds. On further secondary examination, her chest had air entry bilaterally with a high pitch wheeze and some stridor on auscultation. There was clear respiratory distress with rapid shallow breathing, nasal flaring, tracheal tug and subcostal recession.

1 **What is the differential diagnosis?**

A Respiratory symptoms:
- Asthma.
- Anaphylaxis.
- Foreign body.
- Pulmonary embolism.
- Anxiety.

Hypotension:
- Vasovagal attack.

Rash:
- Generalized urticaria.
- With a falling blood pressure can be a sign of infection/sepsis.

2 **How do we differentiate those in Q1?**

A (a) The patient doesn't have a history of asthma or any known allergies that the school are aware of. A foreign body would also produce a **monophonic wheeze** or **stridor**, with possible unilateral lung involvement, depending on where it had lodged.

(b) Her age makes a pulmonary embolism unlikely and she also is not indicating any specific pain.

(c) While anxiety and a foreign body are a possibility, the **erythematous rash** and **angioedema** (swelling) suggest an allergic cause to the respiratory symptoms but if they persisted on treatment, this would be investigated and ruled out in hospital. While the patient has a degree of urticaria, it is more likely to be something more severe causing the respiratory problems.

(d) While the patient has hypotensive symptoms that could be due to a vasovagal attack, it is more likely to be one of the others due to overlapping symptoms.

(e) This patient's temperature was normal and she was systemically well which helps to rule out sepsis.

(f) To differentiate asthma and anaphylaxis, consider the onset of symptoms and also the type of symptoms. Wheeze, difficulty in breathing and respiratory distress could be due to either cause. You would suspect asthma more in cases where the children had been running around (exercise induced), recent respiratory illness or with a history of wheeze. Both asthma and anaphylaxis can have environmental and allergenic triggers.

(g) The severe hypotension, angioedema and an erythematous rash suggest an acute allergic reaction. The sudden onset (likely to be proceeded by feelings of nausea and then closing of airways) would differ from the onset of wheeze only in asthma.

> To **diagnose anaphylaxis**, all three of the following should be present:
>
> - sudden onset of symptoms;
> - life-threatening ABC problems;
> - skin and/or mucosal changes (these can be subtle).
>
> Remember to look out for GI symptoms preceding reaction (Resuscitation Council 2008).

3 **What can trigger an acute allergic reaction?**

A Any allergen specific to the patient can trigger an allergic response. In asthma, these are often exposure to allergenic and environmental triggers such as house dust mite, pets, pollen and viral infection and can occur acutely or even after chronic exposure. Anaphylaxis tends to be due to allergenic triggers such as insect bites, certain foods such as nuts, legumes or a new drug. People with anaphylaxis will generally have had a much milder reaction to their allergen on a previous occasion and then experience more severe reactions on subsequent exposures. Food is the most common cause in children (Alves and Sheikh 2001) but overall insect stings or bites account for 32% of cases (Peng and Jick 2004).

The crew take a more detailed history from the school nurse and begin to put together a management plan. There has been no injury or trauma that preceded the attack. There is no previous anaphylaxis in the school records and the patient does not have asthma. The airway was clear, with no obstruction. The girl has not had any new medications or vaccinations given at school. While Sadie wasn't eating when the incident occured, the playground monitor mentions that she was sharing some food with one of her friends that looked like a cereal bar.

Anaphylaxis is defined as a severe, life-threatening, generalized or systemic hypersensitivity reaction (Johansson et al. 2003).

While the school are attempting to speak to Sadie's parents, the crew begin on a management plan. While they are not absolutely sure she is having an anaphylactic reaction, it is safest to treat as such if it is suspected and then treat for asthma if the treatment fails (see Figure 17.1).

Supportive treatment is started and Sadie is given 50% oxygen via a Venturi mask at a flow rate of 12 L per minute. As the crew suspected a reaction of some form, they decided to administer adrenaline and prepare a neb of salbutamol as well. Sadie continues to be hypotensive so they give a bolus of fluid, i.v.

Adrenaline 1:1000 is the primary treatment for anaphylaxis with no contraindications for use in an emergency (Simmons 2009).

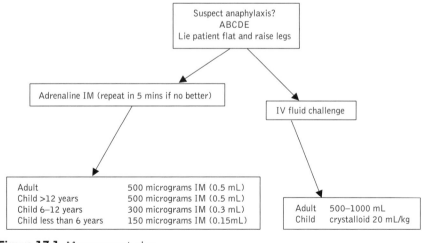

Figure 17.1 Management plan

Source: Adapted from Resuscitation Council 2008.

4 **What happens in the immune system during an anaphylactic reaction?**

A An anaphylactic reaction is known as a Type 1 reaction in that it produces an immediate response on exposure to allergen (usually 5–10 minutes). It is IgE mediated and causes sudden massive release of antihistamine from mast cells and also causes release of inflammatory cells such as cytokines into the bloodstream to defend against the allergen 'invader'. This produces the sudden hypotension, angioedema and shortness of breath as the airways constrict. Some people are thought to be genetically predisposed to react this way to certain triggers, making them atopic. The fall in blood pressure compromises blood supply to internal organs and so must be reversed using adrenaline 1:1000. The dose is repeated if necessary at five-minute intervals according to blood pressure, pulse and respiratory function.

5 **How does adrenaline work?**

A Adrenaline is an **adrenoceptor agonist** which works on smooth muscle to help constrict blood vessels. This helps to improve the blood pressure. It also helps to relax the muscles in the lungs to reduce the bronchoconstriction. The patient might need more than one dose to improve their symptoms.

6 **Why must the patient be referred straight to the emergency department?**

A Biphasic anaphylaxis is the recurrence of symptoms within 72 hours with no further exposure to the allergen. It occurs in between 1–20% of cases depending on the study examined (Lieberman 2005). It should be managed in the same manner as anaphylaxis (Simmons 2009).

Key learning points

- Adrenaline is the first line treatment in suspected anaphylaxis.
- The patient might decide they feel better after treatment and refuse to go to hospital. The adrenaline might only have a short-term effect in anaphylaxis and there is always the risk of secondary attacks. Therefore, prompt transfer to the ED is still important.
- An autoinjection pen (EpiPen) is normally provided by the hospital or GP for self-administration should another attack occur.
- Future exposure to that same allergen (things like nuts or pollen that you can be allergic to) will trigger this allergic response again.

REFERENCES

Alves, B. and Sheikh, A. (2001) Age specific aetiology of anaphylaxis. *Arch Dis Child* 85(4): 348.

Johansson, S.G., Bieber, T., Dahl, R., Friedmann, P.S., Lanier, B.Q. and Lockey, R.F. (2003) Revised nomenclature for allergy for global use: report of the Nomenclature Review Committee of the World Allergy Organization, October 2003. *J Allergy Clin Immunol.* 113(5): 832–6.

Lieberman, P. (2005) Biphasic anaphylactic reactions. *Ann Allergy Asthma Immunol.* 95(3): 217–26.

Peng, M. and Jick, J.A. (2004) Population-based study of the incidence, cause, and severity of anaphylaxis in the United Kingdom. *Arch Intern Med.* 164: 317–19.

Resuscitation Council (2008) *Emergency Treatment of Anaphylactic Reactions: Guidelines for Healthcare Providers*. Available at: http://www.resus.org.uk/pages/reaction.pdf

Simmons, F.E. (2009) Anaphylaxis: recent advances in assessment and treatment. *J Allergy Clin Immunol.* 124(4): 625–36.

Case outline

Nadia is a healthcare assistant who visited Imran, a 78-year-old man who has lived alone since his wife died four years previously and had been suffering from dementia for the last three years. He doesn't recognize her when she goes over to say good morning and seems confused and drowsy. With a full glass of water next to him, it is clear he has had nothing to drink overnight and is very dry, finding it difficult to speak with dry, cracked lips. Concerned that he might be very unwell, she calls for an ambulance.

The paramedics arrive at Imran's home 10 minutes later, expecting to see a generally unwell elderly man. They go into the home to speak to Imran; it is clear he is confused (Nadia claims this is more pronounced than normal) and is finding it difficult to form clear sentences due to his dry mouth. While trying to talk, he begins to cough, revealing a deep rattling cough which produces some green phlegm. It is clear that the crew are going to have great difficulty gaining a clear history from Imran so begin observations while questioning Nadia.

Bystanders

A third party history can be invaluable when a patient is unable to be clear due to age, mental state or conscious level. This doesn't necessarily have to be from a relative; the care worker here will have a good idea about what is normal for this patient and also know his medical and drug history.

Baseline observations

Response:	patient is confused and agitated, looking pale and clammy;
Airway:	dry and clear with poor air entry;
Breathing:	RR 24 bpm with prominent rattle to his cough;
Circulation:	HR 110 bpm full heart sounds are normal;
Blood Pressure:	90/58 mmHg;
ECG:	tachycardia but no obvious abnormalities present;
Disability:	GCS of 15;
Exposure:	crackles pronounced in right lung field;
Glucose:	BM 4.5 mmol/L
Temperature:	39.1°C, urine dipstick (from the catheter bag) shows no signs of infection;
SpO$_2$ sats:	81% (on air).

Imran has had a reduced appetite and claims he does not like the food he has been given, despite it being similar to what he has always eaten. He normally takes fluids well, apart from the last 24 hours where he seems increasingly dry. He has a permanent urinary catheter due to an enlarged prostate restricting the urethra but when Nadia went to change the catheter bag this morning, there was only 10 ml of fluid (over the last 12 hours) whereas he usually produces between 50 ml and 150 ml overnight.

His current medication includes:

- antibiotics (amoxicillin) for the chest infection;
- blood pressure-controlling tablets × 2;
- antidepressants;
- inhalers for COPD, which has only been recently diagnosed;
- home oxygen for when he is feeling breathless.

Imran is normally coherent and only suffers with mild dementia at this point and depression for which he sees his GP. He suffers with regular coughs and colds and is an ex-smoker, giving up after his wife died from lung cancer.

On examination of the chest, there is poor air entry with prominent **crackles** heard throughout the right lung fields. Heart sounds are normal, with no additional sounds and an ECG shows a tachycardic patient but with no significant abnormalities.

1 **What is the differential diagnosis?**

A • Infection and possible sepsis with a significantly high temperature and tachycardia. The patient is likely to be hypovolaemic with the reduced urine output and this is confirmed by marked hypotension. The fact that he has dry mucosal membranes and has not been drinking any water further proves this concern. Any vomiting or diarrhoea should also be excluded as this further loss of fluid can impact on the severity of the patient's fluid imbalance.

• Respiratory tract or a urinary tract infection (UTI). Confusion in the elderly is a classic sign of infection. UTI has been excluded by urine dipstick finding no positive signs of protein, blood or leukocytes/nitrates. The chest sounds and low oxygen saturations (81%) point towards a respiratory tract pathology such as a chest infection or pneumonia. However, other causes of infection will be ruled out once he gets to the hospital. The fact the patient also suffers with COPD will make him more susceptible to chest infections as well.

• Changes in consciousness levels or signs of recent confusion in the elderly indicate that they should have their blood sugar checked for deranged glucose control. This could simply be due to a reduced food intake or be a marker of diabetes. The fact that Imran hasn't been eating as much recently (if at all in the last 24 hours) would be a possibility to consider if his blood sugar was low. His blood glucose is normal (4.5 mmol/L) and this rules out any hypoglycaemic cause for his confusion.

2 **What are the key risk factors for pneumonia?**

A • **Immobility:** you are less likely to be able to clear secretions while there is a reduced ability to fight any infection.

- **Age:** the very young or the elderly are most susceptible to pneumonia.
- **Smoking:** this can exacerbate the situation.
- **Ongoing lung pathology:** asthma or COPD where there is increased production of lung secretions and reduced clearance alongside a weaker immune ability to fight infection given the comorbidities.

After examination and evaluation of risk factors, the ambulance crew decide that Imran will need to be taken to hospital. His observations confirm that he is unwell with a possible infection, which will need hospital investigation. The crew, however, grow increasingly concerned as Imran becomes more confused, refusing to allow the paramedics to transfer him to the trolley-bed yet still consenting to be taken to hospital. He then becomes unable to tell the crew where he is and still doesn't recognize Nadia, who is now very concerned about his state, saying she has never seen him like this before.

Second set of observations

Response:	patient remains confused and agitated;
Airway:	dry and clear;
Breathing:	RR 28 bpm, raised by 4 bpm;
Circulation:	HR 120 bpm, up by 10 bpm;
Blood Pressure:	88/55 mmHg. This second reading is lower than before;
Disability:	GCS of 15;
Temperature:	39.2°C;
SpO$_2$ sats:	86%, now on oxygen (2 L nasal).

3 **What is your immediate management strategy?**

A) Imran is still talking to you and despite the respiratory rate, his airway remains patent. If any additional help is required due to reducing consciousness you should support by placing an airway. Oxygen remains to correct the oxygen saturation and help reduce his respiratory rate to a more comfortable level. With his heart rate climbing and his hypotension worsening, concerns over the risks of hypovolaemic hypotension (such as hypoxic damage to internal organs) mean that fluid resuscitation should be initiated immediately. A large-bore cannula is inserted into the left arm and a bolus of 0.9% saline given to improve the blood pressure and also correct the fluid imbalance from his dehydration.

   If in a more rural location, where transfer to hospital will take a significant length of time, consider initiating antibiotic treatment but supportive treatment is your main priority. Antibiotics are ideally given within the first hour (Kumar et al. 2006) but with blood cultures taken prior to antibiotic administration to determine organism involved and their sensitivity to various antibiotic treatments.

4 **Why is the lactate level raised in sepsis?**

A) Anaerobic respiration occurs in this septic state and so lactate begins to accumulate (this is usually cleared by aerobic respiration). A lactate level of more than 4 mmol/L is thought to indicate tissue hypoxia, and should be addressed.

5 **Why do blood cultures need to be taken?**

A Blood cultures enable the causative organism to be identified and to define the sensitivity of the organism to different antibiotics. This means that correct antibiotics are given, enabling more targeted therapy and reducing unnecessary prescribing. While this is something that is dealt with in hospital and cultures are not an immediate test, without them it is very difficult to narrow down the bacteria involved at a later stage.

6 **Occurrences of sepsis in pre-hospital care?**

A 27% of ITU admissions in the UK are due to severe sepsis (Harrison et al. 2006) and its current mortality rate remains high at 44%. The plan is currently set to reduce this mortality rate by 25% (Slade et al. 2003). While this will require changes to inpatient management of sepsis in ITU, part of this process also lies in the pre-hospital care of patients from their diagnosis to their rapid transfer to an appropriate ED which offers an opportunity to improve the outcome for patients by providing the following:

> **Sepsis scoring (CRB-65)**
>
> - **C**onfusion (new).
> - **R**espiratory rate (≥30 bpm), (not on beta blockers).
> - **B**lood pressure (systolic <90 mmHg or diastolic ≤60 mmHg).
> - Age ≥**65** yrs.

- Sepsis scoring to screen patients en route to hospital known as the CRB-65 score based on confusion, respiratory rate (≥30 bpm), blood pressure (systolic value <90 mmHg or diastolic value ≤60 mmHg) and age (≥65 yrs).
- Oxygen to maintain O_2 sats at 94% or more.
- Fluid challenge bolus of 300–500 ml colloid and 500–1000 ml crystalloid.
- Re-assess patient between each bolus for signs of improvement or deterioration. These can be repeated twice but at three boluses more specialist intervention is required in the hospital setting.
- Alert the receiving hospital if the patient is in severe septic shock and deteriorating to allow more efficient triage and preparation to occur, all of which leads to better outcomes for very ill patients.
- Antibiotic administration within one hour, ideally following taking blood culture samples.

Key learning points

- Sepsis onset can be rapid, with children and the elderly being most at risk of having a simple infection cause them severe illness.
- The immediate treatment they receive in the pre-hospital setting impacts the likely outcome for the patient.
- The main focus for management is in supportive treatment to stabilize the patient for hospital investigation of underlying cause (i.e. blood cultures, imaging etc.).
- Giving antibiotics may be appropriate if transfer to hospital is likely to be lengthy (always check with your employers clinical policy as these can vary).

REFERENCES

Harrison, D.A., Welch, C.A. and Eddleston, J.M. (2006) The epidemiology of severe sepsis in England, Wales and Northern Ireland, 1996 to 2004: secondary analysis of a high quality clinical database, the ICNARC Case Mix Programme Database. *Critical Care* 10: R42.

Kumar, A., Roberts, D. and Wood, K. (2006) Duration of hypotension before initiation of effective anti-microbial therapy is the determinant of survival in human septic shock. *Critical Care Medicine* 34: 589–96.

Slade, E., Tamber, P.S. and Vincent, J.L. (2003) The Surviving Sepsis Campaign: raising awareness to reduce mortality. *Critical Care* 7: 1–2.

CASE STUDY 19
Market forces

Case outline

The crew are heading back to the ambulance base, when they are flagged down by a market trader who has run from a side street. He tells them his friend is in pain and that he thinks he's having a heart attack.

The crew can't drive the vehicle down the side street as it is full of market stalls, so one of the paramedics grabs the response bag (including a defib.) and tells their colleague to let control know they've got a running call.

The paramedic follows the market trader about 20 metres through the busy pedestrianized street to a stall. A man in his 30s is seated and a small crowd is gathered around. It appears a safe enough scene to approach, but the paramedic first tells the friend to go back and bring the crewmate to the scene so that they don't get separated.

1 | **What are the dangers of getting separated at scene?**

A | On arrival, if the patient is in a serious condition or indeed in need of resuscitation the back-up is delayed. Taking the defibrillator to the scene every single time reduces the risk of getting caught out. Crews should use their experience from the moment the ambulance stops to start assessing a scene and the environment, not just the clinical needs of a patient.

Medical problems in a street setting during the day are inherently less risky than a trauma or a violent event inside a building. Many front line ambulance services flag up addresses where previous calls have caused concern to the crew and a database is kept as a trigger to alert crews of raised risks.

> Asking questions to the patient not only allows the paramedic to assess alertness but also if the patient is relaxed, breathing and conscious, you can safely say that they have a reasonable airway and can continue to assess critical features such as breathing rate and pulse. Time criticality is established, the patient is responding to the paramedic's voice and so she asks what seems to be the problem.
>
> The patient, Sanjay, replies that his chest hurts and he thinks he is having a heart attack. He is clearly short of breath and appears to be anxious and in pain but well enough to hold himself upright in the chair. The paramedic begins a calm assessment of the patient while the second paramedic arrives on scene.
>
> The paramedic begins by taking a pulse, assessing its rate and rhythm and also the breathing rate at the same time. These can be completed together over 30 seconds but

when you are not in a time-critical situation, take your time to ensure you are not rushing and missing anything important.

Baseline observations

Appearance:	pale sweaty and slight cyanosis on lips;
Response:	patient is conscious and in pain;
Airway:	dry and clear;
Breathing:	RR 20 bpm with some external muscular usage;
Circulation:	HR 110 bpm and irregular;
Blood Pressure:	178/110 mmHg
ECG:	tachycardia but no obvious abnormalities present;
Disability:	GCS of 15;
Exposure:	crackles pronounced in right lung field;
Glucose:	BM 4.9 mmol/L
Temperature:	36.9°C;
SpO$_2$ sats:	81% on air.

The paramedic's colleague arrives and gets the person accompanying the patient to write his full name and address down. The paramedic also establishes the patient is regularly attending Dr Shah's surgery in the high street. Sanjay is 38 years old, of Bengali origin, living close by and working full time on the market.

Observations of the patient's face include nasal flaring, mouth breathing, general pallor and slight sweating but experience tells the paramedic that while she should be concerned, the patient doesn't look seriously unwell.

The paramedic continues some questions to establish the cause of Sanjay's pain.

2 **What questions do you need to ask about the pain?**

- When did the pain start?
- What type of pain is it? Can you describe the pain to me?
- How long have you had the pain for?
- Please could you point to the area of the pain?
- What were you doing when the pain came on?
- What has helped relieve the pain?
- Have you ever had symptoms like this before?
- On a scale of 1–10 what level of pain is there?

The best way to approach questions about pain is to be systematic and make sure you don't ask leading questions, make sure the patient's descriptions are their own. By saying, 'is it a crushing pain?' the patient might simple agree with you as they want to say the right thing but can mislead your diagnosis and initial management. While this patient believes he is having a heart attack, he might not be. Any sort of chest pain can be very worrying to patients and their panic over whether or not it is a heart attack can be misleading.

3　**What else might you want to know?**

A　Pre-hospital cardiac conditions, such as angina, previous heart attacks or long-standing arrhythmias can all be related to the current symptoms and can give you a likelihood of this being a repeat episode.

Any family history? While they might not be diagnosed with a heart problem, they may have a relevant family history (e.g. father died of heart attack aged 52).

What tablets do you take? The patient might not know their diagnosis but medication can indicate if they have hypertension, **hypercholesterolaemia**, atrial fibrillation or a clotting disorder; all relevant risk factors for heart disease.

General medical health? Smoking, alcohol intake, obesity and ethnicity also play a role but these will not be questions to focus on in the acute setting. You can always ask these if appropriate or ask a family member.

4　**Can we make a definitive diagnosis yet?**

A　No, he has a set of symptoms that point towards an acute cardiac problem or cardiac episode but as an ECG hasn't been carried out yet, you cannot narrow down the diagnosis further. Since his primary survey showed no significant emergencies, you would suspect one of the following:

- acute coronary syndrome (ACS);
- massive pulmonary embolus;
- dissection of the thoracic aorta;
- tension pneumothorax.

Acute coronary syndrome refers to the presence of an acute myocardial ischaemic state and is an umbrella term used to describe unstable angina, NSTEMI and STEMI. Even though he is not in severe pain, the patient may still be having a heart attack. While crushing pain is the most common onset, some people only experience nausea, sweating and shortness of breath (e.g. diabetics) so a full 12-lead ECG is the best tool for diagnosis. The symptoms are also similar to unstable angina (i.e. pain at any time, even at rest). Knowing what he was doing at the time when the pain came on might also point towards angina, especially if he was physically active or stressed. Your investigations now will be to determine whether it is acute coronary syndrome or pain from another cause. All of the above possibilities are serious conditions and would require immediate transfer to the nearest ED.

> The paramedic sets up the ECG, dials in the age of the patient into the monitor and asks the patient to sit very still while a tracing is taken. The only positive finding on the ECG is a mild ST elevation in leads II, III and aVF (inferior leads) of 1–2 mm. His systolic blood pressure is well over 90 and is high enough to handle glyceryl trinitrate (GTN), and after checking that the patient is not taking sildenafil (Viagra), a single dose of 400 mcg spray is administered under the patient's tongue, followed by 300 mg of aspirin. A repeat ECG is taken a few minutes later after some further history taking, and oxygen is administered via a NRB, to reduce the hypoxia and cyanosis.

The Bengali gentleman is 38 years of age and was unloading some stock from the van to his market stall. The load was heavy and he was out of breath. He stopped when he started to feel some pain in his chest, though he continued after it went away and the pain returned when he started to work again. He decided to stop and his cousin got a chair for him to sit on but after 10 minutes' rest he was still in pain. He was very pale and cold and clammy and he could hear his heartbeat in his head. He was worried so he asked for his cousin to call 999. From the history, the paramedic decides the pain is not **pleuritic** in nature as it is continuous and not linked to inspiration of breath. The patient has now been experiencing the constant pain for a total of 20 minutes (stable angina is pain lasting less than 15 mins, resolving on rest), and describes the pain as central, heavy and radiating up into his neck and shoulder.

Acute coronary syndrome
- Unstable angina.
- NSTEMI (non-ST elevation MI).
- STEMI (ST elevation MI).

5 **What is your diagnosis and why?**

A Pain that starts with effort and is relieved by rest is indicative of angina. If the pain stayed we might consider it muscular, from the lifting, or acute coronary syndrome. The fact that the pain was relieved by rest and was precipitated again by activity points us towards angina (either stable or unstable) as does his history of similar chest pain. The fact it is not resolving after 20 minutes' rest is concerning. The ECG initially pointed towards an ST elevation MI but these changes can also be seen in angina (during pain). The fact that the pain responded well to GTN spray and the ECG changes were transient, reversing on resolution of the pain is more indicative of angina and makes you less concerned about myocardial infarction. However, not all heart attacks have ST elevation and you must weigh up the patient's symptoms and their ECG changes together. Either way, this patient should still be rapidly referred to ED as further investigation is needed to confirm the cause of chest pain and a hospital is a better environment for the patient should the pain reoccur.

6 **How does GTN relieve the symptoms of chest pain?**

A GTN causes vasodilatation (enlargement of the patient's veins). This in turn causes the blood to pool and reduce the pre-load upon the heart. In all, the workload of the heart is reduced and so reduces the oxygen requirement. It is the inability of the vasculature to supply oxygen to the heart muscle that leads to ischaemia and the associated pain so improving flow and reducing ischaemia produces positive effects. It is wise to tell the patient that GTN can cause a headache as one of the side effects.

7 **What other medications might you give a patient in acute chest pain?**

A **Aspirin** in a 300 mg dose has an antiplatelet action which reduces clot formation, along with being analgesic, anti-pyretic and anti-inflammatory. The essential thing is to check against any contraindications such as gastric or duodenal ulcers. Encourage the patient to chew the tablet well so that the powder is absorbed faster in the gut.

8   **In the ambulance, what do you need to do while conveying to the ED?**

A   You'll need to repeat all of the basic observations to look for any changes and monitor for repetition of symptoms or deterioration of his medical condition. A repeat ECG will confirm the reversal of symptoms and give an accurate picture on handover. Be ready to quickly present the ECG on handover, including the findings on the initial, symptomatic version. Gain his latest pain score, further GTN (another 400 mcgs) can be offered if required. If the patient remains in pain then a cannula might need to be sited in the patient's arm and morphine is an option.

> ## Key learning points
> - Acute coronary syndrome covers a variety of acute cardiac problems, all of which are considered as emergencies.
> - The ECG can show transient change so repeat ECGs are useful to both monitor and diagnose.
> - Always balance an ECG result with clinical judgement. MIs may or may not show ST elevation changes and ST elevation doesn't always mean an MI.

FURTHER READING

Morris, F., Edhouse, J. Brady, W. and Camm, J. (2009) *ABC of Clinical Electrocardiography*. London: BMJ Books.

Case outline

A 25-year-old woman, named Carol, complains of abnormal bleeding from her vagina with severe pain. She tells the crew that she has had what seemed like a normal period that started two days ago but the period pain is much worse than normal and has now become a sharp stabbing pain in her pelvis. As she has never experienced anything like this before, she panicked and called an ambulance. She keeps apologizing to the crew for calling them out.

More detail about the pain shows that it came on about 36 hours before, starting as a dull ache, similar to the period pain she used to experience before using the coil. She took pain relief (ibuprofen) and it didn't seem to help at all, in fact, it is much worse now and has become stabbing in nature. She points to the pain being in the left iliac fossa and has not moved or radiated anywhere different.

In terms of the bleeding, she thought she was just having another period but the blood is darker than normal and not very heavy. She also says she doubts she is pregnant as she uses the coil for contraception and has not had sex for at least five weeks. She has also recently split up with her boyfriend about a month ago, explaining why she has been stressed; this is what she attributes the irregularity of her periods to. Otherwise, she claims to be generally well with no other symptoms.

Baseline observations

General appearance:	patient is very anxious and in pain, looking pale and clammy;
Airway:	patent and clear;
Breathing:	RR 18 bpm;
Circulation:	110 bpm, regular in character;
Blood pressure:	130/70 mmHg;
Disability:	GCS 15;
Exposure:	Pupils PEARRL;
Glucose:	BM 7.1 mmol/L
Temperature:	36.4°C;
SpO$_2$:	96% on air.

On examination of the abdomen, there is no obvious swelling but she is very tender in the left iliac fossa. Her pain score is 8/10.

1   **What could this area of pain relate to?**

A   (a) Normal menstrual bleeding +/– **endometriosis**. Vaginal bleeding can be normal if part of the menstrual cycle. The pain this patient is experiencing could be the pain associated with that, especially if she suffers with a condition called endometriosis which can cause more severe pain and heavy bleeding. These patients, however, would experience this on every cycle. The normal symptoms can be masked by the use of IUD (intrauterine device such as the coil) or oral contraceptive pills as they both disrupt normal hormone balance and are used to control these symptoms on a regular basis.

(b) Ectopic pregnancy. Any abdominal pain in a sexually active female should be assumed an ectopic pregnancy. While mortality rates for ectopic pregnancies are falling, it still remains the highest cause of mortality in the first trimester of pregnancy and so poses a huge risk to the patient if the diagnosis is missed.

(c) Miscarriage. The patient may not yet know they are pregnant but can present in a similar way to an ectopic pregnancy. Bleeding is generally lighter and may present as spotting rather than profuse bleeding. Pain is more cramp-like over the lower abdomen or lower back. As with all presentations, symptoms can vary case-to-case and the message to take home is to assume ectopic pregnancy until proven otherwise by further investigation in hospital.

Also ...

Cancers of the vagina or cervix can also present with bleeding but are less likely to be associated with acute pain. Also consider that the blood may not be vaginal in origin and may be due to a GI problem. **Haemorrhoids** associated with constipation might be one cause or also consider inflammatory bowel disease causing bleeding into the stools. You might think the patient would know the difference but don't discount it yet.

2   **What are the risk factors for ectopic pregnancy?**

A   Previous gynaecological surgery or infection in the pelvis (e.g. pelvic inflammatory disease or sexually transmitted infection such as Chlamydia) can create scar tissue. This scar tissue makes migration of the embryo more difficult or causes it to attempt to implant in the wrong place. Any damage to the fallopian tubes or structural abnormality can cause ectopic pregnancies.

> An **ectopic pregnancy** is when the products of conception implant outside the endometrial cavity. The current incidence for ectopic pregnancies is at around 11.1 in every 1000 (CEMACH 2007).

Previous ectopic pregnancies can also pose a risk.

IUD, (Mirena coil or copper coil) work by preventing implantation of the embryo into the endometrium. While it is contraceptive, if for some reason pregnancy does occur, the risk of ectopic pregnancy is increased to 1/20 (NICE 2011). Smaller risks include smoking, increased age and multiple sexual partners.

3   **Can this patient be pregnant if she has a contraceptive device fitted?**

A   IUDs don't last forever and are replaced periodically, normally every 3–5 years. If this patient is due a new device, it might have failed and not be providing her with contraceptive cover. Women who use IUDs for the control of heavy/painful bleeding might have a return of their symptoms when the device expires and this also contributes to the differential diagnosis. There is also always the risk that an IUD has been expelled or dislodged which will affect its function.

The paramedic asks Carol again if there is any risk of her being pregnant. The patient says that she hopes not as she split up with her long-term boyfriend about a month ago and has started seeing someone new.

On further questioning it becomes clear that Carol's IUD was fitted about four years ago. She hadn't thought about having a new one fitted as she was out of the habit of having to think about contraception. She has also not been using any other forms of additional contraception with her new partner (increasing her risk of sexually transmitted infections).

Second set of observations

General appearance:	the patient is less anxious but remains in pain;
Airway:	patent and clear;
Breathing:	RR 16 bpm;
Circulation:	90 bpm and regular;
Blood pressure:	130/70 mmHg;
Disability:	GCS 15;
Exposure:	pupils PEARRL;
Glucose:	BM 7.2 mmol/L
Temperature:	36.5°C;
SpO$_2$:	96% on air.

---

4 **What is an ectopic pregnancy?**

A An ectopic pregnancy is a pregnancy outside the uterine cavity with the majority being in the fallopian tube but they can also occur in the cervix, ovary or extra-uterine (i.e. in the abdominal cavity).

5 **What is the management plan?**

A If Carol were acutely unwell with signs of shock (hypotension, tachycardic) rapid transfer to the nearest ED would be required. Resuscitate with IV fluids if required to maintain BP above 90 systolic and stabilize on the way to hospital.

As Carol is haemodynamically stable, she can be fully examined and referred on to the emergency department where she can undergo a pelvic examination. Continue to monitor closely as ectopic pregnancies can rupture and increase risk to the patient.

Pain and bleeding in early pregnancy occur in about 1 in 5 clinically confirmed pregnancies. In 50–60% of these the pregnancy will continue and will have a successful outcome ('threatened miscarriage') but the symptoms may indicate impending miscarriage (25–30%) or ectopic pregnancy (10–15%) (NICE 2011).

The crew should:

- start two IVs and prepare the patient for immediate transportation to the emergency department. Should haemorrhage occur she will require blood transfusion on arrival and might require emergency surgery. Currently, there is insufficient evidence of significant haemorrhage. Her pulse is slow and steady, even with postural changes;
- convey to hospital as she might have an ectopic pregnancy. While you cannot be sure, the safest thing for the patient is to transfer her where further investigations will be carried out;
- continue with further history and examination en route if there has not been opportunity to ask already. Details about gynaecological history and the features discussed above will all aid in evaluating the cause for the symptoms for ED team at handover.

6 **What investigations will be completed at hospital?**

A A pregnancy test will be carried out to confirm whether or not Carol is pregnant. A positive test will then lead to the team wanting to perform an ultrasound to try and find the source of the ectopic (if there is one) or the location of the implanted embryo. Ectopic pregnancy is usually diagnosed using a transvaginal (internal) ultrasound but sometimes the pregnancy is so early on that it is not visible or is not found. Management options include both medical and surgical options. An injection of methotrexate (which kills and helps with the removal of the cells of the embryo) is used medically and **hCG** levels are monitored to see if the treatment has worked or not. Sometimes no treatment is given at all as some ectopics do resolve themselves. The patients do require careful monitoring, though. The most invasive option is surgical removal of the tube or tissue involved.

Key learning points

- In cases of abdominal pain in women of reproductive age, you must always be suspicious of ectopic pregnancy.
- Symptoms of ectopic pregnancy can vary, a typical picture doesn't always occur.
- Ectopic pregnancy is considered an emergency as risk of rupture is high and mortality can occur.

> Between 2003 and 2005 there were 10 **deaths** from ectopic pregnancy in the UK, giving a maternal mortality rate of 0.4 per 1000 women who become pregnant.
> Two thirds of these were associated with substandard care (NICE 2011).

REFERENCES

CEMACH (2007) *Confidential Enquiry into Maternal and Child Health: Saving Mothers' Life. Reviewing Maternal Deaths to Make Motherhood Safer: 2003–2005*. Available at: http://www.cemach.org.uk

NICE (2011) *Pain and Bleeding in Pregnancy*. Available at: http://www.nice.org.uk/nicemedia/live/12342/50042/50042.pdf

CASE STUDY 21
To be or not to be

Case outline

Winter coughs and colds strike at us all, indeed both crew members in this case study had recently had colds and were still troubled by persistent coughs. When control dispatches the next 'job' on the Tetra handset, the crews head for the vehicle. Starting the engine and pushing the green active and mobile button, the call shows up to be a persistent cough. The crew responds professionally in the direction of the city centre but can't help commenting en route that they are about to attend a 999 call to a cough when both crew members already have one.

1 **Why do some ambulance crews resent attending low-priority calls?**

A The training and development of modern crews involves years of academic and clinical development. Call rates have risen year on year and the excess demands placed upon health emergency services is disproportionate to the resources now available. It is likely this crew have not had a break and are working back-to-back cases when they don't feel 100 per cent. Excess pressure from managers usually means staff avoid taking sick days.

The only information they have about the patient before arrival from the update screen, is that his name is Ajay, he is 57 years old and he has been increasingly unwell with this cough over the last week. On arrival, the crew walk into a small end of terrace, welcomed by the patient's wife and taken into the living room. Ajay is lying on the sofa, clearly unwell and sweating profusely.

Brief questioning, mainly answered by Ajay's eldest son as both the parents speak very limited English, tells the crew that he has had the cough for the last couple of weeks but has been really unwell over the last few days. The cough is productive with both green and rust coloured sputum. The main reason the family decided to call for an ambulance is because he started coughing up a small amount of blood last night and again this morning. He has had a fever on and off for nearly a week now but mostly finds he wakes up in the middle of the night drenched in sweat.

Ajay has only been back in the country for the last three weeks, having just been on a two-month trip to see family in Mumbai. He noticed that he was unwell as soon as he returned home but was used to picking up infections from travelling and expected it to resolve on its own as it always did. A family member in Mumbai was also suffering with a cough and he assumed he caught it off him. He has noticed that the cough has progressively got worse (was initially a dry tickly cough) and he has lost his appetite. He has lost some weight but puts this down to not eating as normal.

While the technician takes baseline observations the paramedic continues his questioning.

Baseline observations

Airway:	patent and clear;
Breathing:	RR 36 bpm;
Circulation:	regular but raised at 128 bpm;
Blood pressure:	186/98 mmHg;
Disability:	GCS 15;
Exposure:	Pupils PEARRL;
Glucose:	BM 3.5 mmol/L;
Temperature:	38.4°C;
SpO$_2$:	92% on a non-rebreathing mask;
ECG:	12-lead shows no abnormality.

Inspection of the patient's chest showed clear use of accessory muscles and taking out the stethoscope and carrying out auscultation exposed a deep crackle in the bases and he was clearly struggling. Listening to the chest is an art that is often underperformed by many ambulance crews. Taking the opportunity to listen to relatively healthy chests can assist when one gets the opportunity to actually listen to signs of disease.

The crew asks the son about the patient's general health and if he has suffered with any other illnesses. He was able to explain that he had no obvious illness other than he'd been told to ease up on his diet after he had developed late onset diabetes three years previously. His heart was strong and his own doctor in India was attempting to lower his **cholesterol** using statins that he was purchasing via the internet.

The crew, knowing he'd recently flown into the UK, were slightly concerned this could be a disease of tropical origin but this is thrown into confusion as Ajay has now been back in the country for nearly three weeks. The fact that none of the other family members were showing signs of the symptoms in the last three weeks suggests that it might not be too contagious. Ajay doesn't smoke (and never has) and doesn't suffer with asthma or any other chronic lung disease that may be the reason for his cough. The obvious bloodstaining in the **haemoptysis** was concerning. He has not vomited at all and has had no diarrhoea. Breathing was tired and fast in between the bout of coughs and had a distinct rattle to it.

> **Haemoptysis**
> Coughing up blood (of respiratory origin).

2 **What might be causing his symptoms?**

A The symptoms point towards this being an infection. The fever (temp. of 38.4°C), along with the cough and the examination of the chest, suggests a chest infection. The two things you are concerned about in an unwell person (as this gentleman is), are TB and pneumonia. Both are generally caused by bacterial infection where the disease has spread via tiny droplets of saliva from the coughs or sneezes of the primary infected person. Both respiratory diseases tend to affect those with a weaker immune system (young, old and immunocompromised) but can occur in anyone.

   The other thing to consider in this case given his symptoms is lung cancer. Weight loss and loss of appetite are both red flag signs for possible cancer. The fact that he has also had haemoptysis is another poor sign as is a persistent cough that is not resolving on its own. The fact that he has never smoked makes a diagnosis of lung cancer less likely but it is still a possibility. Further investigation will be needed in hospital.

3 **If it is an infective cause, does this man have TB or pneumonia?**

A Table 21.1 gives us some clues as to the cause of Ajay's symptoms.

Table 21.1 A checklist of TB vs pneumonia symptoms

Checklist	TB	Pneumonia
Pathogen	Mycobacterium tuberculosis	Multiple pathogens (viral, bacterial or fungal). *Strep. pneumoniae* is most common
Onset	Slow progressing, can also be reactivated from previous infection	Can be acute in onset or can develop
Cough	Productive, may have haemoptysis, chronic (>3 weeks)	Productive cough not resolving, may also have haemoptysis
Fever	Yes, worse at night (night sweats)	Continuous fever
Systemic symptoms	Weight loss, pallor, fatigue	Weight loss, joint and muscle aches
Examination of chest	Can be normal. Auscultation may show crackles in apical region	Can be normal. Auscultation may show crackles over infected area (lung bases)
Associated disease	Immunosuppresion, very young or very old	Chronic respiratory disease, immunosuppresed, young or old
Social factors	Associated with foreign travel to endemic regions, primary contact, overcrowding and poverty, more likely in inner-city areas	Associated with smoking and immobility (unable to clear lung secretions)

There is a great deal of overlap between these conditions but a few features are more suggestive of TB. Ajay has had recent foreign travel (Mumbai is an endemic area for TB), he has had a possible contact and also has night sweats. His other symptoms can be attributed to either disease.

4 **Is the patient likely to be infectious?**

A Too difficult to say at this stage, but more than likely, and universal protection has to be considered against airborne particulates. Use a mask, gloves and perhaps an apron if available. After the call a thorough disinfection of all kit that came into contact with Ajay would be wise. TB is an infectious disease and patients are advised to avoid contact with others susceptible to the disease (i.e. immunocompromised) for two weeks after initiating treatment.

The balance between not alarming the patient and the family and protecting the crew are a difficult wire to traverse over the general care and compassion for the patient who is clearly quite unwell. Ideally, crews don't wish to catch any illness and take it home to their own family and as such ambulance crews have good access to occupational health to ensure they have all the relevant boosters. TB generally only affects those who are immunocompromised or close regular contacts of the person infected.

The crew were advised that the patient had a persistent cough, but had initially considered it low risk and probably the same cough and cold that they had. The crew were informed several days later that Ajay had in fact been suffering with TB. He might, however, have had the disease for several months or even have a reactivation of a previous unknown infection.

5 **Why should crews be concerned about TB? Surely it is a rare disease?**

A The **WHO** (2010a, 2010b) tells us that there were 9.4 million new cases of TB in 2009 with 1.7 million people dying of the disease in the same year. However, mortality rates are falling and more people than ever are being successfully treated. While it is mainly a disease of the developing world, cities (such as London) are seeing a rise in cases again due to immigration, travel and living conditions. TB is more commonly seen in immunocompromised patients, especially in HIV, and with the incidence of HIV rising, we are seeing more HIV-associated TB. Parts of the world known to have higher rates of TB include Africa, South East Asia, parts of Europe and Central America.

6 **How should the patient be managed now?**

A This is not an emergency but Ajay is clearly unwell and TB will require hospital investigation. Treatment will then be initiated once the diagnosis is confirmed and Ajay's contacts will be tested and may require treatment as well. As the paramedics treating this patient, the best thing you can do is to phone ahead and inform the hospital you have a patient with suspected TB. He will require isolation on arrival and the more notice you give the emergency department, the more time they have to logistically prepare to receive the patient.

7 **What is the prognosis for Ajay?**

A Treatment of TB is very effective and involves giving four different antibiotics (**isoniazid, rifampicin, pyrazinamide**, and **ethambutol**) over a period of 6–9 months. He must take his medication for the complete amount of time, as missing doses can result in production of resistant strains of the bacterium which then don't respond to further treatment, making his illness much worse.

Sometimes, the body is able to build a protective barrier around the focus of the infection and the disease becomes latent but can go on to reactivate at any stage.

TB can reactivate outside of the lungs in other organs, such as the kidneys, bone and lymph nodes. Patients with HIV tend to present in an atypical way and can easily present with extrapulmonary TB in the first instance. HIV-related TB is more difficult to treat and is often associated with a poorer prognosis.

Key learning points

- Patients with suspected TB require isolation in hospital so warn the hospital you are travelling to that you have a suspected TB patient to give them time to prepare.
- TB is more common in those with underlying problems with their immune system (e.g. HIV), the very young and the elderly.

REFERENCES

World Health Organization (2010a) *Global Tuberculosis Control: Epidemiology, Strategy, Financing.* Available at: http://www.who.int/tb/en/

World Health Organization (2010b) *Tuberculosis Global Facts 2010/2011.* Available at: http://www.who.int/tb/publications

The rise and fall of Gladys Jones

Case outline

'Fall, query, assist' is not what you want to hear with 45 minutes of your shift remaining.

In this instance the crew responded promptly but as it was a low-category call it didn't require lights and sirens. Kit choice at this stage is relatively simple: primary response pack (including a defib.), an oxygen barrel bag with bag valve mask (BVM) and an aspirator. Falls are a common element of 999 calls and the elderly make up a high percentage of this. A combination of poor mobility and, on occasions, too many small trip hazards makes this a regular call-out.

Gladys Jones was known to the crew; they had also attended last week on nights to help her back into bed after her alarm cord had been pulled by the bedside. Gladys on that occasion had missed the edge of the bed after returning from the toilet and had slid to the floor and without her walker she had no possibility of hauling herself up. The crew had checked her over and, with Gladys stating that this happened all the time, they left her at home and arranged for the warden to call in at breakfast when the home help arrived to double-check all was still OK.

On this occasion, Gladys was lying face down in the kitchen, having slipped on a wet floor after she had accidently kicked the cat's drinking bowl over. While she always uses her walker when leaving the house, she likes to try and get around on her own in the house.

Gladys was conscious and moaning that she wanted to get up as she had been lying there for hours. The crew placed a blanket over her and got down to inspect her while trying to ask pertinent questions to establish what had happened.

Baseline observations

Airway:	good, with her dentures still in place;
Breathing:	RR 30 bpm and shallow (lying on floor);
Circulation:	regular at 108 bpm;
Blood pressure:	110/75 mmHg;
Disability:	GCS 15;
Exposure:	Pupils PEARRL, size 4;
Glucose:	BM 7.5 mmol/L;
Temperature:	36.5°C;
SpO$_2$:	94% on air, 96% on a nasal cannula.

A small cut on the bridge of the nose had swollen up but it was not bleeding at this stage. She also mentioned that her left hand hurt as she had reached out when she fell.

1   **What are the key priorities in the initial management plan?**

A   Once the collar is on log-roll her over to examine the front and relieve her breathing. Airway is clear but the shallow rapid breathing as she is bearing weight on her chest on the floor is not an ideal situation. Respiratory rate of 30 bpm is above the upper boundaries of normal but she is lucid, coherent and not cyanosed, the SpO_2 indicates oxygen saturation of 94%.

Complete a secondary survey on her back. Secondary surveys don't normally start on the back but after checking for cervical spine issues and applying a collar, it would be wise to quickly check the thoracic and lumbar vertebrae and pelvis before continuing.

Board her under suspected C-spine injury after a fall. Cervical spine injury is always a possibility but Gladys hasn't fallen from a height as she slipped over and broke some of her fall with her left hand, which is slightly swollen. However, the cut to the bridge of the nose leaves the crew considering that her head also took some of the force of the fall.

Stand Gladys up and see how she is on her feet, though best not on this occasion as the crew have no idea what is actually happening and could miss some serious underlying problem in their haste to clear down from this call. She is clearly a regular faller and might have an underlying problem leading to her falls.

2   **What are the important risk factors for having a fall?**

A   • **Polypharmacy:** there is a linear relationship between the number of medications a patient takes and their risk of falling (Ziere et al. 2006).
   • The number of drugs a patient takes is likely to be related to underlying **chronic disease** (another risk factor in recurrent falls), with circulatory disease, arthritis, COPD and depression most associated (Lawlor et al. 2003).

There was no need to cut any clothing off to reveal any potential underlying issues. The collar was not easy to size or apply in this position and so, using their experience, the crew fitted a collar that appeared to be the most appropriate and decided to re-check it when the patient was turned.

Utilizing the warden and a relative visiting the flat of her neighbour opposite, the crew directed the extra help to turn Gladys on to the rescue board. The experienced paramedic led the procedure and held the collared neck and head in the 180-degree manoeuvre. Re-positioning her midline onto the board was relatively easy as Gladys was of small build, weighing no more than 50 kg.

Gladys at this point was keen to sit up and had to be persuaded to stay still for her own benefit. This didn't go down very well as she was convinced a cup of tea and a rest in her chair would resolve everything. Indeed, she was quite reluctant about the plan to take her to the ED for an X-ray of the wrist and to treat her cut nose. It was also likely that the doctors would want to check for any underlying medical conditions once she was at the hospital.

3 **How can the crew rule out stroke, diabetes and heart disease using the secondary survey?**

A
- **FAST** test was negative. Glucose of 7.5 mmol/L (breakfast eaten around an hour ago).
- The 12-lead ECG was NSTEMI but did show an irregular rhythm with some atrial flutter.
- Her BP remained stable for the two readings taken with her lying down (110/76 and 108/75).
- She showed no obvious signs of dehydration; however, she admitted she was not drinking as much, as she was fed up going to the toilet as often as she did. This of course might be a factor of the recent falls at night.

The crew put a simple non-adhesive dressing on Gladys's nose and held that down with two small strips of hypoallergenic tape just to give a covering. When asked about what medications she takes regularly, Gladys points to the table in the living room, showing a large dosette box with all her medications divided up. There was also a long list written next to the box with instructions to help Gladys remember when to take them all. The warden

Falls are the leading cause of mortality resulting from injury in people aged >75 in the UK. Furthermore, more than 400,000 older people in England attend ED following an accident (NICE 2004).

also helps by keeping a log and a record booklet of daily visits, a useful source to check ongoing care and any recent occurrences that perhaps Gladys didn't remember.

Three years before Gladys fractured the neck of her femur in a trip in the rear yard hanging out clothing when she overreached and tumbled. The home help now assists in this area, but Gladys often feels like her life is no longer hers and everyone is doing and deciding for her.

Communication is everything at this stage and the need for empathy to support Gladys in what is an emotionally traumatic situation must not be forgotten or underestimated. The feelings related to loss of control and the potential loss of independence are major factors in older patients refusing to go to hospital. Time might be required to explain why they need to go to hospital and to remind them that all decisions regarding their care are their own.

People like Gladys are the best calls because they test you on every level, clinically, emotionally and, probably top of the list, with real care. The opportunity to talk to Gladys on the way to the hospital allowed the crew to build a good rapport and at the same time find out a little about her. This also had the added benefit of relieving some of her stress by taking her mind off going to hospital.

Further assessments to re-check baseline observations while chatting en route are conducted in an unhurried matter. At the hospital the crew handed her over to the nursing Sister on triage who directed them to a side examination room.

4 **Should the crew remove the collar and board? Or leave Gladys as she is?**

A The obvious thing is to leave well alone until an X-ray or at least until given release by the attending medical staff at ED. Kit can be picked up later by the oncoming crew and a note on the PRF and on the driver's seat also helps the messages to and from oncoming crews.

Sometimes the nursing and medical staff ask the crew to stay behind and assist with the undressing of a patient if they are above-average size and weight, but there is a significant pressure placed on the crew by EOC to turn the call round in 15 minutes from arrival including all paperwork to reduce the 'job-cycle' and keep the vehicle available for the next call waiting.

5 **How can further falls be prevented for Gladys?**

A Patients with recurrent falls or a problem with their gait are offered a falls risk assessment at home following referral from paramedics at scene. The falls assessment team looks at both hazards in the home and potential problems with health (such as vision and cognitive impairment) to find solutions. Examples include a medication review to see if any of the current prescriptions interfere with balance, strength and balance training and addressing trip hazards in the home. Patients at risk of falling may also need fracture risk assessment and **osteoporosis** checks so that, should they fall, treatment can be given to reduce fracture risk. NICE (2004) guidelines describe a pathway of assessment and intervention to prevent falls in the elderly.

> Up to 14,000 people die annually in the UK as a result of an osteoporotic hip fracture (NSF, 2001). It is clear that falling has an impact on quality of life, health and health care costs (NICE 2011).

Key learning points

- While some elderly patients who fall can be picked up and placed back in bed or in a chair, there are often underlying problems causing them to fall. A falls assessment can help address the reasons behind this.
- Be patient, falling is very distressing as is being taken to hospital, so take time to explain what is happening to the patient.
- Ask the patient exactly what they remember about falling and if they experienced any symptoms before or as they fell. In case they forget this later, it can be helpful to have this documented straight after the event.

REFERENCES

Lawlor, D.A., Patel, R. and Ebrahim, S. (2003) Association between falls in elderly women and chronic diseases and drug use: cross sectional study. *BMJ* 327(7417): 712–27.

NICE (2011) *The Assessment and Prevention of Falls in Older People*. Available at: www.nice.org.uk/nicemedia/live/10956/29585/29585.pdf.

NSF (2001) *National Service Framework for Older People*. Department of Health, London.

Ziere, G., Dieleman, J.P. and Hofman, A. (2006) Polypharmacy and falls in the middle age and elderly population. *Br J Clin Pharmacol*. 61(2): 218–23.

FURTHER READING

Audit Commision (1997) *The Coming of Age: Improving Care Services for Older People*. National Services Framework. Department of Health, London.

Tinetti, M.E. (2003) Clinical practice: Preventing falls in elderly persons. *N Engl J Med*. 348(1): 42–9.

Case outline

Every ambulance crew has areas that when they are called to give rise to heightened expectation. The bypass on the north of town is one that has had more than its fair share of serious road traffic collisions (RTC).

Depending on traffic conditions, time of day and so on, the scene can indicate several aspects of the seriousness of the situation and, in particular, the mechanisms of injury. The oncoming traffic on this occasion was non-existent, indicating perhaps the traffic collision had occluded the road in both directions, just like a blocked artery.

The call had been dispatched to the crew as 'car versus lorry' and it was clear as they were pulling up it would be wise for the driver of the ambulance to U-turn the ambulance to give better **egress** if they needed to leave the situation speedily, this being dependant on the time criticality of the injuries.

A compact size four-door car was wedged under the rear section of an articulated lorry that had been making a wide swing into a narrow entrance. The lorry driver was standing by his cab smoking a cigarette and looking concerned about the incident.

The car had three occupants. A driver and two passengers: one in the front seat and one in the rear. Because the car was positioned partly under the lorry trailer it was not easy to accurately see the condition of all the occupants of the car; however, the driver's door was partly open and a bystander was holding the driver's head.

1 **What are your first considerations?**

A **Safety**

Where is the ambulance positioned (fend off and egress) and have the ambulance crew members donned full personal protective equipment (PPE)? Leave the emergency warning lights on to clarify to approaching motorists and other emergency vehicles where the scene is. The fire service had immobilized the car to ensure that it wouldn't move unnecessarily during the removal of the patients. They were attempting to reduce risk of fire by cutting the battery supply. The engine had been turned off and the keys removed and placed upon the car dashboard.

Mechanism of injury

The risk of c-spine injury was already being dealt with by the bystander, and the other passengers appeared to be unconscious, both with serious head injuries. It is common to approach the front of the car to gain the visual and auditory connection with the occupants. That was not possible this time due to the lorry.

Resources

Do you need more resources (police, fire and ambulance including helicopter and/or doctor)? The driver of the ambulance crew contacted the emergency operations centre and asked for two further ambulances. There were up to four potential patients and the extra hands will be extremely useful during the extrication and in the conveyance of patients to the ED or trauma unit.

2 **Could you have missed any other patients?**

A This singular incident had no other vehicles or pedestrians involved and it had been witnessed by three other cars waiting behind the rear of the lorry that had slowed down considerably to make the difficult right turn into a small lane. The car had overtaken these cars at an excessive and dangerous speed and collided in to the rear unloaded trailer lorry as it turned.

Police were also on scene and starting to cone off the scene to ensure that any evidence was safely protected from excess and unwanted foot and tyre traffic. They will also mark final stopping points of all vehicles. Further police cars had been dispatched to each end of the bypass to stop any further road traffic using the road until the situation was stabilized and under full control.

The crew was able, with fire service assistance, to open the doors on the off-side of the vehicle. On approach to the first passenger in the front seat, it quickly became clear that she was dead, with massive chest and head injuries. That corner of the car had made significant contact with the lorry that intruded into the passenger side, crushing the young girl of around 15 or 16 years of age.

> **Youth fatalities**
> In 2009, 65 young people aged under 15 were killed and 18,307 were injured on the roads in the UK, 2267 of them seriously (Department for Transport 2010a).

The rear passenger was unconscious, with serious head injuries. He had no seatbelt on and might have been thrown forward into the passenger and bounced back on to the rear seat. The driver of the car, who was fully conscious and not complaining of any injuries, had a collar fitted by the attending paramedic who asked the bystander to remain holding the head.

The focus had now shifted to dealing with the rear passenger while awaiting further assistance.

3 **Do any of the baseline observations for the rear passenger give concern?**

Response:	unresponsive;
Airway:	clear of any blood or fluids;
Breathing:	RR 14 bpm and shallow (lying on floor);
Circulation:	120 bpm at the carotid artery;
Blood pressure:	96/48 mmHg;
Disability:	GCS 3;
Exposure:	Pupils PEARRL, size 4;
Glucose:	BM 8.7 mmol/L;
Temperature:	36.8°C;
SpO$_2$:	95% on a nasal cannula.

A Although there was a clear head injury it wouldn't be considered to be catastrophic haemorrhage. This low BP can't be attributed to the head injury and so a neck-to-knees prior to the secondary survey was undertaken to discover that the young adolescent male, around 16 years old, had bilateral fractured femurs (clear swelling and deformity) and with that significant trauma blood loss could reasonably be expected to be many litres into the tissue. It is important not to miss other significant injuries and so the chest was also examined and found to be clear with equal breaths and nothing significant found in these cramped conditions. It is very possible that other injuries associated with high velocity impact might have occurred such as pelvic fracture (another cause for extensive blood pooling) and vertebral damage.

4 **Is this a time-critical extrication from the vehicle?**

A The patient was unconscious (head injury) with low blood pressure (fractured femurs), and was deemed to be time critical and thus met the category for rapid extrication. Fortunately the other two ambulances had arrived and were divided into one crew to assist with the extrication and the other crew to re-check the lorry driver and the driver of the car.

The passenger patient, once collared and assisted onto the spinal rescue board, was head-blocked and strapped while transferred on to the trolley-bed and loaded. There was no room in the vehicle to apply a traction splint and it was decided that it would be dealt with in the vehicle en route, along with initial treatment.

5 **What treatment should occur prior to departure to hospital?**

A Twin lines were placed into the passenger's arms but although fluids were attached it was decided that he would not be infused as the systolic BP was holding steady at this stage. Excess fluids can increase blood pressure but also increase bleeding and the further reduction of the haematocrit (proportion of red blood cells in the blood volume). As the blood pressure is holding at the moment and the extent of any internal bleeding is unknown, it is probably wise to hold off fluids unless there is concern about hypovolaemic shock. Constant re-assessment is continued while on the way to the nearest trauma hospital and an appropriate alert call was placed via control.

> Between 5 and 18% of trauma patients receive fluids (generally crystalloids) representing 9–65 patients/year/population (Dretzke et al. 2004).

The important thing in this patient is to monitor his blood pressure and blood loss (Table 23.1) checking for signs of hypotensive shock. Small amounts of blood loss can show very little difference in signs and symptoms. Mental state can also indicate problems with the patient ranging from normal and alert, anxious or angry to confused and unconscious in severe blood loss. Table 23.1 shows changes in objective signs used to estimate severity of blood loss.

6 **What information do the hospital require on the alert call and on arrival?**

A An alert call will have been placed out to the hospital and on the way the paramedics give the further information that they have a young adult male (unknown name and DOB), adding details of vital signs and any treatment given already. It is also important to mention that the patient is head-blocked onto a spinal rescue board. All this information will help the staff at the ED to adequately prepare to receive an acute trauma patient. Paramedics will hand over

Table 23.1 Evaluating blood loss

Evaluating blood loss				
	Class 1	*Class 2*	*Class 3*	*Class 4*
Blood loss (%)	<15	15–30	30–40	>40
Volume (ml)	750	800–1500	1500–2000	>2000ml
BP	Normal	Normal	Reduced	Very Low
Pulse (bpm)	<120	100–120	120	>120

Source: JRCALC (2006).

the patient on arrival and might be required to assist in moving the patient and answering any initial questions from the medical team, also ensuring that the PRF is complete before leaving the hospital and preparing for the next call.

Outcomes

The driver was breathalyzed and found to have an excess of alcohol in his system; he was arrested and taken into custody. His young girlfriend was declared dead at scene and the fire service took over 40 minutes to cut the car open to extricate her frail body. The lorry driver was also breathalyzed and found to be clear of alcohol or blame for the accident. The scars would stay with him for life. In 2008, 2538 people were killed on British roads (Department for Transport 2010b). While the number of fatalities is declining year on year, it still averages seven deaths per day including car, motorcycle and pedestrian road users.

Key learning points

- Use a similar evaluation approach to all trauma situations as each will be varied and you need to be systematic in order not to miss any parts out.
- Safety.
- Assess scene (JRCALC suggests use of METHANE) and triage patients.
- Any other casualties missed?
- Primary survey (ABCDE).
- Secondary survey (if non-time critical).

METHANE

M – major incident standby or declared

E – exact location of incident

T – type of incident

H – hazards

A – access and egress

N – number, severity and type of casualties

E – emergency services present (more required?)

REFERENCES

Department for Transport (2010a) *Road casualties Great Britain: 2009 Annual Report*. London: The Stationery Office.

Department for Transport (2010b) Fatalities in reported road accidents: 2008. Road Accident Statistics Factsheet No. 2 – 2010. Available at: http://www.dft.gov.uk

Dretzke, J., Sandcock, J., Bayliss, S. and Burls, A. (2004) Clinical effectiveness and cost effectiveness of prehospital intravenous fluids in trauma patients. Available at: http://www.dft.gov.uk

JRCALC (2006) *Clinical Practice Guidelines*. London: ASA.

CASE STUDY 24
Attempted suicide

Case outline

The crew are sent to a 49-year-old man who is threatening to kill himself. Further update information on the mobile data terminal (MDT) states that he is recently divorced and living alone, and his children and ex-wife have moved to another city. He sees no purpose any more in living. His father took his own life, so why shouldn't he? He says that he is sitting on the flat roof of the block of flats that he lives in. The building is 10 stories high and he knows that if he jumps, the fall will kill him. The patient, John, is clearly distressed on the phone but wanting to talk with the dispatcher on the phone because he says he has no one to talk to.

> **Depression** is a major health problem and is now the fourth leading cause of disease burden worldwide (Ustun et al. 2004).

---

1 **Which of the following statements about this patient and his management is NOT true?**

A a This patient is at high risk of successful suicide.

b The dispatcher should attempt to keep the caller on the phone until the crew arrive and can reach him.

c When the crew reach the patient and interview him, they should inquire specifically whether he has made any concrete plans about how he would kill himself.

d If the paramedic team feels that the patient is in real danger of harming himself, they might transport him against his will to the hospital.

Answer (d) is NOT true. The crew will need to get support from an approved social worker or a police officer. Conveying patients against their will is not acceptable.

This patient is at high risk of suicide given his social circumstances, recent life events and his family history.

It is important that someone should stay on the line with the caller until the paramedic team can reach him. This will help prevent him from doing anything irrational in the meantime and also provides someone for the patient to talk to. The fact that he called 999 and asked for the ambulance service indicates that he still has some mixed feelings about killing himself; his telephone call was a plea for help. This contact should not be interrupted once it has begun.

The crew on arrival can talk to the patient and inquire about plans he has made. Generally, the patient who has made concrete plans is more likely to carry them out than a patient who merely expresses a vague desire 'to end it all'. Don't be afraid to ask a patient about suicide and what their plans are, some can be worried about giving the patient ideas but there is little danger of this. It might be a relief for the patient to have someone willing to talk to them about it.

2 **Why is the patient at high risk of suicide?**

A This patient is indeed at high risk of a successful suicide, for he has several significant risk factors:

- he is male (the rate of successful suicide is higher among men than women);
- he is recently divorced. Stressful life events can trigger both depression and increase susceptibility for suicide. Other examples can be grief after the death of a loved one or losing a job;
- he is living alone; those who are isolated are at higher risk;
- he is depressed and sees no point in living any more;
- he has a history of suicide in the family.

Factors which are supportive and protect the patient can be children and family (someone to live for) and religion (either as a source of support or their beliefs condemning suicide).

On arrival, the dispatcher has sent more information on to the MDT after her conversation with John. He says that he has been seeing his GP for the last six months about his mood and has recently started taking an antidepressant, citalopram, but he doesn't think the tablets are working and he just cannot cope anymore. This is the first time he has tried to commit suicide but admits he has been considering it for the last two months, which is why his GP started treatment three weeks ago. He has a history of depression, having seen a counsellor in his early 20s for anxiety problems and low mood. He says his recent symptoms of depression are much worse than then. He says he coped OK when he and his wife divorced but it's the fact that he can't see his children anymore as they've moved away which sent him down this depressive spiral.

So he has not made an attempt to kill himself. Today he hasn't taken any pills or completed any final acts (writing a suicide note or finalizing his will). He says he has been drinking this morning but denies any illicit drug use. When asked what he would do in the future if he didn't commit suicide today or he was unsuccessful, he says he would probably try again if his current mood were still the same.

The safety of the crew

Without overstating the obvious, clearly the crew need to be cautious. The situation is fragile and the patient has not been professionally assessed. So far we have a second-hand account of a phone conversation from the patient to the control centre. In your professional capacity it is vital you consider physical problems and exclude any critical problems relating to the primary survey.

3 **Does the patient have capacity?**

A It is obvious that a patient can be admitted for mental health problems and yet still have full capacity. The fact the patient has a crisis doesn't mean they don't understand what is happening. However, they still might be a risk to themselves or others and so it might be necessary to section the patient if they will not cooperate with care for their own good.

4 **What sort of risk is the patient at?**

A A simple tool called 'Suicide and Self-harm Risk Assessment Form' (Table 24.1) allows us to assess low medium and high risk. The tool is based on the SAD PERSONS Scale (Patterson et al. 1983).

Table 24.1 Suicide and self-harm risk assessment form

Item	Value	Patient score
Sex: Female	0	
Sex: Male	1	1
Age: less than 19 years old	1	
Age: greater than 45 years old	1	1
Depression/hopelessness	1	1
Previous attempts at self-harm	1	
Evidence of excess alcohol/illicit drug use	1	1
Rational thinking absent	1	
Separated/divorced/widowed	1	1
Organized or serious attempt	1	
No close family, or job or active religious affiliation	1	1
Determined to repeat or ambivalent	1	1
Total patient score	–	7

<3 = low risk   3–6 = medium risk   **>6 = high risk**

This patient has a score of 7, showing that he is of high risk.

5 **What help and support is required at the scene?**

A Should it be necessary to get further assistance it is better to consider this in the first 10–15 minutes as there is likely to be a delay in getting a police officer to attend. More often than not a social worker will be involved in this case and might have already been called. Most mental health teams have an on-call crisis team who can assist both in the short term and in the long-term follow-up.

6   **Should the crew update the emergency control of the latest situation?**

A   Delays at scene can drag on and sometimes the patient will change their mind at the last moment and not wish to attend voluntarily, even though most will. Keeping control up to date is helpful and the crew might be relieved by an oncoming crew if shift change occurs. Ideally services prefer to keep the same crew, but that is not always possible.

As they talk to the patient, the crew recognize he is at a reasonably high risk and the driver contacts control via her Tetra handset, asking for an ETA of the patient's approved social worker. Should there be a prolonged delay the crew can then consider if a police officer on site might be a viable option, if one is available.

7   **Can paramedics section a patient?**

A   Laws that govern admission of a patient against their will are covered by the 1983 Mental Health Act (England and Wales) with amendments made in 2007. The current law allows for compulsory admission usually alongside the approved mental health professional (AMHP) and a doctor under a section 4 (2), usually carried out by a doctor who knows the patient well, such as the GP or psychiatrist treating the patient. The law states that the AMHP must have seen the patient in the last 24 hours and that getting the opinion of a second doctor before sectioning would cause too much delay. This distinguishes it from a section 2 where two doctors are required for approval. A close relative may also be involved in this decision. Paramedics are not able to section a patient to force them to hospital against their will.

> **Informal vs formal**
> Of all those admitted to hospital for psychiatric reasons, 90% do so informally. Others are admitted under the Mental Health Act against their will (Doy et al. 2004).

Section 4 allows for the emergency assessment of a patient who is perceived to be a risk to themselves or others. It only lasts for 72 hours so any further assessment or treatment required would need to be completed under a different section. As a general rule, in hospital, a section 2 is used for assessment and a section 3 is for treatment but neither are used in the emergency pre-hospital setting.

Patients can be admitted 'informally' (of their own will). This is either because they have given valid consent or they are unable to give consent and are being treated on the basis of necessity, acting in the patient's 'best interests' or acting under a 'duty of care' as part of the Mental Capacity Act. Remember, though, that patients who have full capacity have the right to refuse treatment (having a mental illness does not remove the patient's capacity).

8   **Where do you transfer the patient to?**

A   If the patient has any medical problems requiring immediate treatment (e.g. cuts or a tablet overdose), take them to the nearest ED. If they require psychiatric treatment, they can be referred to the nearest appropriate centre from there. Many mental health units do not treat medical illness, only psychiatric. If the patient is medically well, take them to the nearest open mental health hospital. Availability of an open emergency walk-in at a mental health unit can be limited at certain times of day so always check ahead. Control can advise.

> ### Key learning points
>
> - Management of patients with depression who are wanting to commit suicide can be difficult. Always ask for support where needed but do not be afraid of making the situation worse.
> - Assess the patient's risk of committing suicide to help in your decision as to whether they need to be transferred to the nearest mental health unit.
> - Always assess for physical illness. Any medical problems that require treatment must be treated in a general hospital.

REFERENCES

Doy, R., Burroughs, D. and Scott, J. (2004) Mental health: consent, the law and depression-management in emergency settings. *Emerg Med J* 22: 279–85.

Patterson, W., Dohn, H., Bird, J. and Patterson, G. (1983) Evaluation of suicidal patients: The SAD PERSONS Scale. *Psychotomaties* 24(4): 343.

Ustun, T.B., Ayuso-Mateos, J.L., Chatterji, S., Mathers, C. and Murray, C.J.L. (2004) Global burden of depressive disorders in the year 2000. *The British Journal of Psychiatry* 184: 386–92.

FURTHER READING

National Institute of Clinical Excellence (NICE) (2004) *Depression: The Management of Depression in Primary and Secondary Care*. Available at: http://www.nice.org.uk

Mental Health Law Online, http://www.mentalhealthlaw.co.uk

CASE STUDY 25
Sickly sweet

Case outline

A 55-year-old American tourist has called the reception of his hotel and asked them for assistance. The hotel decides to call an ambulance as their normal local doctor is not available in the evenings and the gentleman says he feels too unwell to take a taxi to the nearest hospital. A non-urgent call is sent and the crew arrive in good time, carrying their kit up to his room. The patient, Jim Lennon, is accompanied by his wife and complains of a worsening cough and some difficulty in breathing. He has had chronic obstructive pulmonary disease (COPD) since age 50, which is well controlled on his normal combination of inhalers (**salbutamol, salmeterol** and **fluticasone**).

1   **Do paramedics have to treat visitors to the UK?**

A   Emergency care is always provided by the NHS. The ambulance service does not show any favour to UK nationals and treats all patients the same. Modern services have a variety of excellent tools at hand to assist with translating for patients clients and families who do not speak English.

The patient thought he might be getting a chest infection so one week before he had started taking the **prophylactic** antibiotics his doctor in America had sent him on holiday with, and also has started a course of steroids. He doesn't take any nebulizers nor does he need home oxygen. He has been taking his inhalers as normal and his symptoms are not relieved by increasing his dose. Today he has marked **dyspnoea** even when going to the bathroom and he remains concerned about his persistent cough. He also has hypertension which is actually normally poorly controlled using an **ACE inhibitor**, ramipril. His wife also mentions that he has been more confused than normal over the last day or two and has been complaining of feeling very tired. She has also noticed he has been getting up to go to the toilet a lot in the night and has been drinking a lot of water but still seems to be thirsty. The patient has not had any urgency or pain on passing water, simply increased frequency.

Baseline observations

Response: alert;
Airway: clear of any blood or fluids, his lips look dry and cracked and he complains that his mouth is dry, asking for water;

Breathing: RR 28 bpm, he is apyrexial. His lungs are clear with good air entry bilaterally. No accessory muscles are being used and no cyanosis is present;

Circulation: 120 bpm at the carotid artery;

BP: 115/64 mmHg;

Disability: he generally looks pale and fatigued. GCS 15 AVPU;

Exposure: pupils PEARRL, size 4;

Glucose: BM 13.9 mmol/L (250 mg/dL) showing he is hyperglycaemic;

Temperature: 36.8°C;

SpO$_2$:   97% on air.

The patient interjects that he ate a meal delivered by room service around two hours
ago so they are unsure of how representative the results will be. A urine dipstick is
negative for blood, **leucocytes, neutrophils** and **ketones** but is positive for glucose.

2   **What might you suspect from the initial results?**

A   For someone who normally has high blood pressure, the low blood pressure is a concern. Even
though he is on an antihypertensive, the patient has already told you his blood pressure is
normally poorly controlled. The fact that his pulse and respiratory rate are also raised might
make you think that he has an infection or is in sepsis (see Case Study 18). He has mentioned
that he thought he had a chest infection. However, he is already on antibiotics and he is
apyrexial (doesn't have a temperature), making this unlikely. His chest examination and good
oxygen sats suggest that this isn't an exacerbation of his COPD. The main concern here is that
he has been feeling thirsty and urinating more than normal. Given his general appearance, this
might suggest he is dehydrated. The high blood sugar and urine dipstick alongside the dehydrated state could point towards diabetes mellitus.

3   **What are some of the reasons why Mr Lennon's blood sugar is high?**

A   High blood sugar (hyperglycaemia) can be caused
by both type I and type II diabetes mellitus. It can
also be caused by impaired glucose intolerance,
where there is reduced sensitivity to insulin so,
despite normal insulin release, glucose isn't metabo-
lized as quickly, increasing circulating levels. Some
drugs can have the side effect of causing raised
blood glucose, such as some antipsychotic drugs.
Blood glucose can also release in times of severe
illness (e.g. sepsis) or chronic inflammation.

> Diabetes mellitus is a metabolic
> disorder characterized by
> chronic hyperglycaemia with
> disturbances of carbohydrate, fat
> and protein metabolism resulting
> from defects in insulin secretion,
> insulin action or both.

4   **What defines a patient as diabetic?**

A   The WHO (2003) uses plasma glucose levels to determine whether or not someone has
diabetes:

* fasting plasma glucose: >7.0 mmol/L;
* random plasma glucose: >11.1 mmol/L.

Both results are needed in an asymptomatic individual, but in symptomatic patients, only one result is required.

This patient has symptoms that suggest he is diabetic but the crew can only measure his glucose in pre-hospital care. BM sticks (for measuring glucose) use whole blood, differentiating it from a plasma sample. Levels measured from plasma are generally slightly higher than those seen in BM. While we can say this patient has current hyperglycaemia, further investigation is needed for diagnosis.

Some patients can have chronically elevated blood glucose but not high enough levels to diagnose them as diabetic. This means that the person has impaired glucose intolerance and has a high risk of going on to develop type II diabetes mellitus. A further test, called a glucose tolerance test, is used to diagnose this.

> **Diabetes** is a common life-long health condition. There are 2.8 million people diagnosed with diabetes in the UK and an estimated 850,000 people who have the condition but don't know it (Diabetes UK 2011).

The crew ask more questions relating to his health background and any underlying medical conditions. His family practitioner had told him a random blood glucose was high so he completed a glucose tolerance test and had his **hbA1c** tested a few days before he went on holiday but hasn't received the results yet. While he is not grossly overweight now (with a BMI of 27.8), he hasn't always been in good shape. He has lost about two stone in weight over the last six months on the advice of his doctor because of his family history of type II diabetes and coronary heart disease. He says that losing the weight has also helped him control his blood pressure. He also used to smoke 25 cigarettes a day but quit three months ago with the help of nicotine patches, which he still uses. He drinks socially, about 25 units per week, and uses no recreational drugs. Mr Lennon works in IT in California and says he came to England to relax after recent health problems.

The crew are concerned about the high blood glucose but they do not carry insulin so cannot do anything about it acutely. The best course of action is to take Mr Lennon to the nearest ED. The only immediate intervention the crew should consider is to reverse the patient's dehydration. A large-bore cannula is placed in the patients left arm and he is given a bolus of saline. The hyperglycaemia will require blood tests in hospital. It would also be wise to take an ECG, even though he complains of no chest symptoms. Diabetics can suffer with painless MIs due to damage to their nerve function. Reassurance is important in this case as well. He is clearly feeling short of breath and may be worried about an exacerbation of his COPD, especially being in a foreign country with the thought of needing to travel home. While it is always important to maintain good communication with patients, sometimes you need to remind patients that they are in good hands and relieve any unfounded worries they have. This case has the potential to be complicated given the range of symptoms, the vague timeline and his comorbidities.

5 **What are some of the potential complications of hyperglycaemia?**

A Acutely, ketoacidosis can occur. This is generally seen in type I diabetes where a patient doesn't produce enough insulin and ketones are produced in an alternative glucose metabolism. This leads to a dangerous acidotic state, diabetic ketoacidosis, and requires emergency transfer to hospital. In cases where insulin is present, you can have a **hyperosmolar** hyperglycaemic non-ketotic coma. This is a serious metabolic illness where there is marked hyperglycaemia, severe dehydration but no sign of ketosis (overly sweet smelly breath, ketone positive on urine dipstick). This again requires emergency transfer to hospital for more intensive management. Chronically high levels of blood sugar can lead to vascular disease, most commonly resulting in kidney damage, heart disease and nerve damage.

6 **How might steroids be contributing to his blood glucose level?**

A Steroids interfere with normal glucose metabolism, leading to hyperglycaemia. This works by increasing hepatic glucose production and release but also reducing the ability for insulin to stimulate glucose uptake, leading to overall increase in blood glucose levels. Hyperglycaemia induced by **corticosteroids** can have a mild effect on fasting blood glucose levels but exaggerates postprandial blood glucose elevations.

7 **How should treatment in diabetes compensate for this?**

A If a patient uses diet control for their diabetes, you would consider giving an oral anti-diabetic agent or adding in pre-prandial short-acting insulin for the duration of use of the steroids. If they are already using insulin to control the diabetes, their treatment regimen might need to change to accommodate this.

In this case, Mr Lennon is likely to have a high glucose level during the peak dose of his steroids. It is also likely that his blood glucose levels will drop if he rapidly drops the prednisone dose.

8 **What other drugs must you be cautious of in diabetics?**

A There are a number of other drugs that can alter glucose metabolism, causing blood levels to go up or down.

Thiazide diuretics in high doses can cause blood glucose levels to go up as can **beta-blockers**. This doesn't occur in all patients and might simply affect insulin sensitivity rather than directly increasing glucose. **Salbutamol** (or Ventolin) tablets can also affect glucose metabolism. **Phenytoin** (or Dilantin) tablets are often prescribed for epilepsy and can cause an increase in blood glucose levels.

Some people take **MAO inhibitors** for psychiatric illnesses. MAO inhibitors make sulphonylurea tablets (used to treat diabetes) work more strongly and alter blood sugar. In the same way, some antibiotics such as **chloramphenicol, tetracycline** and **sulphonamides** can cause sulphonylurea medication to have a stronger effect. If patients go onto these tablets they need to monitor their glucose levels more often. Taking insulin or sulphonylurea tablets with alcohol can lead to a low blood glucose level and so patients are advised to drink in moderation.

> **Key learning points**
> - Diabetes can be a hidden disease that patients are unaware they have until they have complications. National screening programmes help to reduce this.
> - Hyperglycaemia doesn't always mean the patient has diabetes; there are a number of different causes including chronic illness.
> - Diabetes has a number of complications, both acute and long term, making blood sugar control vital to diabetic patients.

REFERENCES

Diabetes UK (2011) *Introduction to Diabetes*. Available at: http://www.diabetes.org.uk/Guide-to-diabetes/Introduction-to-diabetes/What_is_diabetes/

World Health Organization (WHO) (2003) *Screening for Type 2 Diabetes*. Available at: http://www.who.int/diabetes/publications/en/screening_mnc03.pdf

Glossary

4Hs and 4Ts

- Hypovolaemia – a lack of blood volume.
- Hyperkalaemia or hypokalaemia – both excess and inadequate potassium can be life threatening.
- Hypothermia – a low core body temperature.
- Hypoglycaemia or hyperglycaemia – low or high blood glucose.
- Cardiac tamponade – fluid building around the heart.
- Tension pneumothorax – a collapsed lung.
- Thrombosis (myocardial infarction) – heart attack.
- Thromboembolism (pulmonary embolism) – a blood clot in the lung.

8 Minute (Orcon): Operational Research CONsultancy was developed by a UK consultancy company in 1974 as a standard for monitoring ambulance service performance.

999 Call: used to summon assistance from the three main emergency services, the police, fire brigade and ambulance, or more specialist services such as the coastguard and, in relevant areas, mountain and cave rescue. Calls to 999 are free. Calls to the European Union standard emergency number 112 are automatically routed to 999 operators.

Access: the entry point to the incident as opposed to the exit point which is referred to as egress.

ACE inhibitor: a class (group) of drugs that are used in the treatment of various disorders correctly named as Angiotensin Converting Enzyme Inhibitors – which is usually shortened to ACE inhibitors.

Acidosis: a condition in which there is excessive acid in the body fluids. It is the opposite of alkalosis (a condition in which there is excessive base in the body fluids).

Adrenaline: a natural stimulant made in the adrenal gland of the kidney. It is carried in the bloodstream and affects the autonomous nervous system, which controls functions such as the heart rate, dilation of the pupils, and secretion of sweat and saliva.

Adrenoceptor (β-agonists): these bind to β-receptors on cardiac and smooth muscle tissues. They also have important actions in other tissues, especially bronchial smooth muscle (relaxation), the liver (stimulate glycogenolysis) and kidneys (stimulate renin release).

Alkalosis: a condition in which the body fluids have excess base (alkali). This is the opposite of excess acid (acidosis).

Allergen: the substance that causes an allergic response is known as an allergen. It contains protein, and almost anything can be an allergen for someone.

Allopurinol: a drug used primarily to treat hyperuricaemia (excess uric acid in blood plasma) and its complications, including chronic gout.

Ambulance: the term *ambulance* comes from the Latin word *ambulare*, meaning to walk or move about which is a reference to early medical care where patients were moved by lifting or wheeling. The word originally meant a moving hospital, which follows an army in its movements.

Amiodarone: an antiarrhythmic agent that is used to treat ventricular arrhythmias and atrial fibrillation.

Amlodipine: a long-acting calcium channel blocker (dihydropyride class) used as an anti-hypertensive and in the treatment of angina. Like other calcium channel blockers, amlodipine acts by relaxing the smooth muscle in the arterial wall, decreasing total peripheral resistance and hence reducing blood pressure; in angina it increases blood flow to the heart muscle.

Anaerobes: these bacteria, called anaerobes, normally live in the GI tract, where there is only a limited amount of oxygen. By definition, the term *anaerobic* means 'life without air'.

Anaphylaxis: an acute multi-system severe type I hypersensitivity allergic reaction.

Angioedema: a swelling, similar to hives, but the swelling is beneath the skin rather than on the surface. Hives are often called welts. They are a surface swelling. It is also possible to have angioedema without hives.

Angiotensin II: a very potent chemical that causes muscles surrounding blood vessels to contract, thereby narrowing blood vessels. This narrowing increases the pressure within the vessels and can cause hypertension. There are medications that block the action of angiotensin II by preventing it from binding to angiotensin II receptors on blood vessels. As a result, blood vessels dilate and blood pressure is reduced. Reduced blood pressure makes it easier for the heart to pump blood and can improve heart failure.

Aniscoria: unequal size of the pupils.

Anticardiolipin: the Anticardiolipin Antibody Syndrome (Lupus Anticoagulant) is caused by an antibody response against phospholipid (a major component of the cell wall). The antibody response results in a heterogenous group of clinical conditions including blood clots, stroke, heart attack, low platelet count, spontaneous abortions, and vague neurologic symptoms.

Anticoagulant: a substance that prevents coagulation; that is, it stops blood from clotting.

Aphasia: a disorder caused by damage to the parts of the brain that control language.

Arrhythmias: a disorder of the heart rate (pulse) or heart rhythm, such as beating too fast (tachycardia), too slow (bradycardia), or irregularly.

Arterial blood gas: is a test that measures the arterial oxygen tension (PaO_2), carbon dioxide tension ($PaCO_2$), and acidity (pH).

Arteriopath: an impairment of the structure or function of the blood vessels which carry blood away from the heart.

Ascites: excess fluid in the space between the tissues lining the abdomen and abdominal organs (the peritoneal cavity).

Asherman seal: allows paramedics and first response personnel to eliminate unwanted air in the pleural cavity and prevent it from re-entering.

ASHICE:
- **A**ge – patient's age.
- **S**ex – whether the patient is male or female.
- **H**istory – what has happened, e.g. patient involved in a front impact RTC with a stationary vehicle at approx 20 mph.
- **I**njuries sustained – maxillofacial, chest, abdomen, possible internal injuries.

- **C**ondition – patient's vital signs i.e. B P, pulse, respirations, O_2 saturation, G C S, R T S. Is the patient cannulated, intubated and any medications given to patient, e.g. oxygen, aspirin, G T N?
- **E**stimated time of arrival to hospital.

Aspirin: also known as acetylsalicylic acid is a salicylate drug, often used as an analgesic to relieve minor aches and pains. Aspirin also has an antiplatelet effect by inhibiting the production of thromboxane, which under normal circumstances binds platelet molecules together to create a patch over damaged walls of blood vessels.

Asymptomatic: a disease is considered asymptomatic if a patient is a carrier of a disease or infection but experiences no symptoms.

Ataxia: the name given to a group of neurological disorders that affect balance, coordination, and speech. There are many different types of ataxia that can affect people in different ways.

Atenolol: a selective β1 receptor antagonist, a drug belonging to the group of beta-blockers – a class of drugs used primarily in cardiovascular diseases.

Atheromatous: an atheroma is an accumulation and swelling in artery walls that is made up of (mostly) macrophage cells, or debris, that contain lipids.

Atony: refers to a muscle that has lost its strength.

Auscultation: the technical term for listening to the internal sounds of the body, usually using a stethoscope.

Bendroflumethiazide: Thiazide diuretic (often referred to as a water tablet) used for hypertension (high blood pressure) and oedema (fluid retention).

Blood pressure: the pressure exerted by circulating blood upon the walls of blood vessels, and is one of the principal vital signs.

Blued in: an expression used by crews to indicate the increased speed of driving on blue light on the way to the hospital with an accompanying call via control to pre-alert medical staff.

Bradykinin: a peptide that causes blood vessels to dilate (enlarge), and therefore causes blood pressure to lower.

Capillary refill test: the capillary nail refill test is a quick test performed on the nail beds to monitor dehydration and the amount of blood flow to tissue. Ideally the hand is held above the heart.

Carbon monoxide (CO): a colourless, odourless, tasteless, poisonous gas produced by incomplete burning of carbon-based fuels.

Carcinoma: the uncontrolled growth of abnormal cells in the body. Cancerous cells are also called malignant cells.

Cardiopulmonary resuscitation (CPR): Actions include performing chest compressions and rescue breaths on people who are not breathing or their heart is not beating.

Chlamydia: a disease caused by the bacteria Chlamydia trachomatis. It is most commonly sexually transmitted. As many as 1 in 4 men with chlamydia have no symptoms.

Chloramphenicol: a bacteriostatic antimicrobial. It is considered a prototypical broad-spectrum antibiotic, alongside the tetracyclines.

Cholesterol: a waxy steroid of fat that is produced in the liver or intestines. It is used to produce hormones and cell membranes and is transported in blood plasma of all mammals.

Cirrhosis: scarring of the liver and poor liver function as a result of chronic liver disease. Symptoms may develop gradually, or there may be no symptoms.

Clinical record (PRF): records comprehensive, accurate clinical and non-clinical information. It records details about the incident to which an operational response has been made and provides space for recording the care provided to a patient.

Clubbing of nails: occurs when the tips of the fingers enlarge and the nails curve around the fingertips. This condition results from low oxygen levels in your blood and could be a sign of lung disease. Clubbing is also associated with inflammatory bowel disease, cardiovascular disease and liver disease.

CO_2: an odourless, colourless gas formed during respiration and by the decomposition of organic substances.

Coagulopathy: a group of conditions in which there is a problem with the body's blood clotting process. These disorders can lead to heavy and prolonged bleeding after an injury.

Colchicine: a medication used for gout. It is a toxic natural product and secondary metabolite, originally extracted from plants of the genus Colchicum.

Colloid: a substance microscopically dispersed evenly throughout another substance. A colloidal system consists of two separate phases: a *dispersed phase* (or *internal phase*) and a *continuous phase* (or *dispersion medium*). A colloidal system may be solid, liquid, or gaseous.

Comorbidities: diseases or conditions that coexist with a primary disease but also stand on their own as specific diseases.

Computer tomography (CT): also called computerized axial tomography (CAT) scanning, this is a medical imaging procedure that uses X-rays.

Continuous Professional Development (CPD): the means by which members of professional associations maintain, improve and broaden their knowledge and skills and develop the personal qualities required in their professional lives.

Convulsion: a medical condition where body muscles contract and relax rapidly and repeatedly, resulting in an uncontrolled shaking of the body.

Coronary Care Unit (CCU): a hospital ward specialized in the care of patients with heart attacks, unstable angina, cardiac dysrhythmia and various other cardiac conditions that require continuous monitoring and treatment.

Corticosteroids: a class of steroid hormones that are produced in the adrenal cortex.

Crackles: crepitations, or rales are the clicking, rattling, or crackling noises that might be made by one or both lungs of a human with a respiratory disease.

C-Reactive protein: a protein found in the blood, the levels of which rise in response to inflammation. Its physiological role is to bind to phosphocholine expressed on the surface of dead or dying cells and some types of bacteria.

Crepitations: crackles in the lungs – usually heard with a stethoscope. Crepitations can be caused by fluid build up or fibrosis of the lung tissues.

Crohn's Disease: a form of inflammatory bowel disease (IBD). It usually affects the intestines, but may occur anywhere from the mouth to the end of the rectum (anus).

Cushing's triad: a clinical triad variably defined as either hypertension, bradycardia, and irregular respiration, or less commonly as widened pulse.

Cyanosis: the appearance of a blue or purple colouration of the skin or mucous membranes due to the tissues near the skin surface being low on oxygen.

Cyclizine: an antihistamine drug used to treat nausea, vomiting and dizziness associated with motion sickness or vertigo.

D-dimer test: a simple and confirmatory test for disseminated intravascular coagulation that can also indicate when a clot is lysed by thrombolytic therapy.

DEFG: acronym for Don't ever forget glucose, which can follow on from ABC and secondary surveys.

Diazepam (Valium): used to treat anxiety disorders, alcohol withdrawal symptoms, or muscle spasms.

Doctor: a qualified practitioner of medicine; a physician.

Dyskinesia: a movement disorder which consists of effects including diminished voluntary movements and the presence of involuntary movements.

Dyspnoea: may also be less fancifully termed as shortness of breath. In the medical sense, dyspnoea tends to refer to shortness of breath deriving from a medical condition and not caused by excessive exertion. Numerous conditions list dyspnoea as a possible symptom.

Dystonia: a neurological movement disorder, in which sustained muscle contractions cause twisting and repetitive movements or abnormal postures.

Egress: defined as an easy get away from a RTC or a major incident. Avoids being blocked in by other vehicles.

Emergency Department (ED): also known as Accident & Emergency (A&E), Emergency Room (ER), Emergency Ward (EW), or Casualty Department.

Emergency Operations Centre (EOC): a central command and control facility responsible for carrying out the principles of emergency support of ambulance staff and associated functions at a strategic level in an emergency situation, and ensuring the continuity of operation of a variety of organizations.

End tidal CO_2 (EtCO$_2$): monitoring (capnography) is a non-invasive method of determining carbon dioxide levels in intubated and non-intubated patients.

Endocarditis: inflammation of the inside lining of the heart chambers and heart valves (endocardium). Symptoms: abnormal urine colour; chills (common); excessive sweating (common); fatigue; fever (common); joint pain.

Endometriosis: a medical condition in which cells from the lining of the uterus (endometrium) appear and flourish outside the uterine cavity, most commonly on the ovaries.

Entonox: a mix of nitrous oxide 50% and oxygen 50%. This is a medical anaesthesia gas, also commonly known as Nitronox.

Erythematous rash: redness of the skin caused by dilatation and congestion of the capillaries, often a sign of inflammation or infection.

Escharotomy: incision into a burn eschar in order to lessen its pull on the surrounding tissue.

Ethambutol: commonly abbreviated to EMB or simply E, this is a bacteriostatic antimycobacterial drug prescribed to treat tuberculosis.

Extracapsular: pertaining to something outside a capsule, such as the articular capsule of the knee joint.

FAST assessment: requires an assessment of three specific symptoms of stroke.
- **F**acial weakness – can the person smile? Has their mouth or eye drooped?
- **A**rm weakness – can the person raise both arms?
- **S**peech problems – can the person speak clearly and understand what you say?
- **T**ime to call 999.

Fluticasone: a synthetic glucocorticoid. Both the furoate and propionate forms are used as topical anti-inflammatories.

Focal: having or localized centrally at a focus; 'focal point'; 'focal infection'.

General Practitioner (GP): a medical practitioner who treats acute and chronic illnesses and provides preventive care and health education for all ages.

Glasgow Coma Scale (GCS): a reliable and universally comparable way of recording the conscious state of a person.

Gliclazide: stimulates the pancreas gland to produce more insulin hormone, thus lowering blood glucose.

Global overview: the first or the early view of scene by the crew as they formulate initial thoughts considering danger response etc.

Glomerulonephritis: a type of kidney disease in which the part of the kidneys that helps filter waste and fluids from the blood is damaged. A common symptom of glomerulonephritis is blood in the urine.

Glucose: a simple sugar (monosaccharide) and an important carbohydrate in biology. Cells use it as the primary source of energy.

Glyceryl trinitrate (GTN): designed to allow the blood vessels in the body to relax and widen allowing more blood to flow through them. In doing so more oxygen can be carried in the blood and the heart does not have to work so hard to keep up with both the demands of the tissues and the resistance caused by the build-up in the vessels.

Gout: a kind of arthritis that occurs when uric acid builds up in the joints. Acute gout is a painful condition that typically affects one joint. Chronic gout is repeated episodes of pain and inflammation.

Green: this is when an ambulance crew or an ambulance car is available for the next call following release at ED or at scene if not required to convey the patient.

Guidelines (National Clinical): recommendations on the appropriate treatment and care of people with specific diseases and conditions within the NHS.

Haemoptysis: the coughing up of blood originating from the respiratory tract below the level of the larynx.

Haemorrhoids: painful, swollen veins in the lower portion of the rectum or anus. Symptoms of haemorrhoids include anal itching, anal ache or pain, especially while sitting.

hbA1c test: indicates your blood glucose levels for the previous two to three months. The HbA1c measures the amount of glucose that is being carried by the red blood cells in the body.

hCG: a gylcoprotein hormone produced during pregnancy that is made by the developing embryo after conception and later by the placenta.

Heparin sodium injection: a type of medicine called an anticoagulant. It is used to stop blood clots forming within the blood vessels.

Hernia: usually a sac formed by the lining of the abdominal cavity (peritoneum). The sac comes through a hole or weak area in the fascia, the strong layer of the abdominal wall that surrounds the muscle.

Herniation (brain): when brain tissue, cerebrospinal fluid, and blood vessels are moved or pressed away from their usual position inside the skull. Symptoms: cardiac arrest (no pulse), coma, lethargy.

Hypercapnia: occurs when there is too much carbon dioxide in the blood.

Hypercholesterolaemia: the presence of high levels of cholesterol in the blood. It is not a disease but a metabolic derangement that can be caused by many diseases, notably cardio-vascular disease. It is closely related to the terms 'hyperlipidaemia' (elevated levels of lipids in the blood) and 'hyperlipoproteinaemia' (elevated levels of lipoproteins in the blood).

Hyperkalaemia: higher-than-normal levels of potassium in the blood. Hyperkalaemia often has no symptoms. Occasionally, people may have the following symptoms: irregular heartbeat, nausea, slow, weak, or absent pulse.

Hyperosmolar syndrome or diabetic hyperosmolar syndrome: a medical emergency caused by a very high blood glucose level.

Hypertension: abnormally high blood pressure, especially in the arteries ie a reading of 140/90 mm Hg or greater.

Hyperuricaemia: a level of uric acid in the blood that is abnormally high.

Hypoglycaemic: the medical term for a state produced by a lower than normal level of blood glucose.

Hyponatraemia: a metabolic condition in which there is not enough sodium (salt) in the body fluids outside the cells. Common symptoms include: abnormal mental state, confusion, decreased consciousness, hallucinations.

Hypoperfusion: decreased blood flow through an organ, as in hypovolaemic shock; if prolonged, it may result in permanent damage.

Hypothalamus: a portion of the brain that contains a number of small nuclei with a variety of functions.

Hypovolaemia: an emergency condition in which severe blood and fluid loss makes the heart unable to pump enough blood to the body.

Hypoxia: a pathological condition in which the body as a whole (generalized hypoxia) or a region of the body (tissue hypoxia) is deprived of oxygen.

IAPP: **I**nspection-**A**uscultation-**P**ercussion-**P**alpation.

Ibuprofen: a non-steroidal anti-inflammatory drug (NSAID) used for relief of symptoms of arthritis, fever, and as an analgesic (pain reliever).

Idiopathic: an adjective used primarily in medicine meaning arising spontaneously or from an obscure or unknown cause.

Ileo-caecal valve: a sphincter muscle situated at the junction of the small intestine (ileum) and the large intestine.

Intensive Therapy Unit (ITU): a part of the hospital where patients who require very close observation are admitted.

Intracapsular: within a capsule, especially within the capsule of a joint.

Intrauterine device (IUD): a small T-shaped plastic device that is placed in the uterus to prevent pregnancy.

IPPA: **I**nspection-**P**alpation-**P**ercussion-**A**uscultation, an outcome-oriented alternative approach.

Ipratropium bromide: an anticholinergic drug used for the treatment of chronic obstructive pulmonary disease.

Ischaemic: relating to or affected by ischemia ie an inadequate supply of blood to an organ or part, as from an obstructed blood flow.

Isoniazid: also known as isonicotinylhydrazine (INH), this is an organic compound that is the first-line antituberculosis medication in prevention and treatment.

Jaundice: also known as *icterus*. Icteric is an adjective used to describe a yellowish pigmentation of the skin, the conjunctival membranes over the sclerae (whites of the eyes), and other mucous membranes caused by hyperbilirubinaemia (increased levels of bilirubin in the blood).

Ketones: ketone bodies are three water-soluble compounds that are produced as by-products when fatty acids are broken down for energy in the liver and kidney. The presence of ketones in the bloodstream is a common complication of diabetes, which if left untreated can lead to ketoacidosis.

Lactic acid: is mainly produced in muscle cells and red blood cells. It forms when the body breaks down carbohydrates to use for energy during times of low oxygen levels.

Leucocytes (white blood cells): outnumbered by the red blood cells 600 to 1, these cells are spherical in shape and slightly larger than red blood cells.

Lidocaine: is used topically to relieve itching, burning and pain from skin inflammations, injected as a dental anaesthetic or as a local anaesthetic for minor surgery.

Limb leads: four leads placed on the extremities: left and right wrist; left and right ankle. The lead connected to the right ankle is a neutral.

Lucid interval: in emergency medicine, a lucid interval is a temporary improvement in a patient's condition after a traumatic brain injury, after which the condition deteriorates. A lucid interval is especially indicative of an epidural haematoma. An estimated 20 to 50% of patients with epidural haematoma experience such a lucid interval.

Lupus anticoagulant antibodies: also known as lupus antibody, LA, or lupus inhibitors, this is an immunoglobulin that binds to phospholipids and proteins associated with the cell membrane.

Major Trauma Centre: patients with multiple, serious injuries may need to be transferred to a major trauma centre which can handle 250 patients per year as a minimum.

Malrotated bowel: twisting of the intestines (or bowel) caused by abnormal development while a fetus is in utero, which can cause obstruction. Occurs in 1 out of every 500 births in the United States.

MAO inhibitors: Monoamine oxidase inhibitors (MAOIs) are a class of antidepressant drugs prescribed for the treatment of depression.

Mechanism of injury: an important part of history taking when finding out about an injured patient. You can tell a lot about the injury when you can visualize what actually happened.

MedicAlert emblems: registered charity providing bracelets or necklets to identify individuals with hidden medical conditions and allergies.

Metabolic acidosis: a condition in which there is too much acid in the body fluids. Symptoms: most symptoms are caused by the underlying disease or condition that is causing the metabolic acidosis.

Metaclopramide: an antiemetic and gastroprokinetic agent. It is commonly used to treat nausea and vomiting, to facilitate gastric emptying in patients with gastroparesis, and as a treatment for migraine headaches.

Metatarsal-phalangeal joint sprain: an injury to the joint and connective tissue between the foot and one of the toes. When the big toe (1st phalange) is involved, it is known as 'turf toe'.

Mobile Data Terminal (MDT): these are connected wirelessly to a central computer, usually at the control center. They can function instead of or alongside the two-way radio and can be used to pass details of jobs to the crew, and can log the time the crew was mobile to a patient, arrived, and left scene, or fulfill any other computer-based function.

Monophonic wheezes: continuous musical tones that are most commonly heard at end inspiration or early expiration. They occur as a collapsed airway lumen gradually opens during inspiration or gradually closes during expiration. As the airway lumen becomes smaller, the air flow velocity increases resulting in harmonic vibration of the airway wall and thus the musical tonal quality.

Morphine: the most abundant alkaloid found in opium, the dried sap (latex) derived from shallowly slicing the unripe seedpods of the opium, or common or edible, poppy, *Papaver somniferum*.

Naso-gastric (NG) tube: used for feeding and administering drugs and other oral agents such as activated charcoal.

Nephropathy: refers to damage to or disease of the kidney. An older term for this is nephrosis.

Neutrophils: the most common type of white blood cell, comprising about 50–70% of all white blood cells. They are phagocytic, meaning that they can ingest other cells, though they do not survive the act. Neutrophils are the first immune cells to arrive at a site of infection, through a process known as *chemotaxis*.

Newbie: a slang term for a novice or newcomer, or somebody inexperienced in any profession or activity.

NSAIDS (non-steroidal anti-inflammatory drugs): these are usually abbreviated to NSAIDs or NAIDs, but also referred to as non-steroidal anti-inflammatory agents/analgesics.

NSTEMI: non-ST elevation myocardial infarction.

Nurse: a nurse is a health care professional who, in collaboration with other members of a health care team, is responsible for: treatment, safety, and recovery of an acutely or chronically ill individual.

Nystagmus: involuntary eye movement; may refer to: physiologic nystagmus or pathologic nystagmus.

Oedema: a condition that causes too much fluid (mainly water) to accumulate in your body. Any tissue or organ can be affected, particularly the hands, feet and around the eyes.

ORCON standards: these are monitored through key performance indicators.

- *Activation* – all calls should have an ambulance 'activated' within three minutes of the phone being answered. This is usually made up of the control room tasking the crew within one minute, and the crew having a further two minutes to be 'on the road'. This is supposed to be achieved with 95% of calls.
- *Category A* calls, which are calls designated by AMPDS as being immediately life threatening. 75% of calls should receive an initial response within eight minutes (of the operator answering the call) and 95% of calls should receive an initial response within 19 minutes. The performance indicator generated by the ambulance service is expressed as a percentage of how many calls meet this.
- *Category B* calls, which are calls designated by AMPDS as being serious, but not immediately life threatening. 95% of calls should receive an initial response within 19 minutes. The performance indicator generated by the ambulance service is expressed as a percentage of how many calls meet this.

Osteoporosis: a condition characterized by a decrease in the density of bone, decreasing its strength and resulting in fragile bones.

Pallor: a reduced amount of oxyhaemoglobin in skin or mucous membrane resulting in a pale colour. This can be caused by illness, emotional shock or stress.

Palmar erythema: reddening of the palms, especially around the base of the little finger and thumb. A number of medical conditions can cause this clinical sign, such as high blood pressure.

Palpable: etymology: L, *palpare*, to touch gently.

Paracetamol: a pain relieving drug discovered by accident when a similar molecule (acetanilide) was added to a patient's prescription about 100 years ago. Known as acetaminophen in the US and paracetamol in the UK. When mixed with codeine it is sold as *Tylenol*.

Paramedics: provide specialist care and treatment to patients who are either acutely ill or injured. They can administer a range of drugs and carry out certain surgical techniques.

Pathognomonic: a sign or symptom that is so characteristic of a disease that it makes the diagnosis.

PEARRL: pupils equal and round reactive to light.

Peptic ulcer: erosion in the lining of the stomach or the first part of the small intestine, an area called the duodenum. If the peptic ulcer is located in the stomach it is called a gastric ulcer.

Per rectum (PR): Latin for from or by the rectum.

Per vagina (PV): Latin for from or by the vagina.

Peritonitis: spontaneous peritonitis is usually caused by infection of ascites, a collection of fluid in the peritoneal cavity. Secondary peritonitis has several major causes. Bacteria may enter the peritoneum through a hole (perforation) in the gastrointestinal tract.

Phenytoin: commonly used antiepileptic. Phenytoin acts to suppress the abnormal brain activity seen in seizure by reducing electrical conductance among brain cells by stabilizing the inactive state of voltage-gated sodium channels.

Plasma protein: blood proteins, also called serum proteins, are proteins found in blood plasma. Serum total protein in blood is 7g/dl.

Pleural rub: pleural friction rubs are low-pitched, grating, or creaking sounds that occur when inflamed pleural surfaces rub together during respiration.

Pleuritic: pertaining to a condition of pleurisy.

Pneumothorax: a collapsed lung, or pneumothorax, is the collection of air in the space around the lungs. This buildup of air puts pressure on the lung, so it cannot expand as much as it normally does when you take a breath.

Polypharmacy: the use of multiple medications by a patient, especially when too many forms of medication are used by a patient.

Polyphonic wheeze: multiple pitches and tones heard over a variable area of the lungs.

Post-ictal: the altered state of consciousness that a person enters after experiencing a seizure. It usually lasts between 5 and 30 minutes.

Pre-alert: the same as a blue call or blued in. Contacting the receiving hospital via EOC to ensure they are made aware of the case to help them prepare for its arrival.

Prokinetic: a gastroprokinetic agent, gastrokinetic, or prokinetic, is a type of drug which enhances gastrointestinal motility by increasing the frequency of contractions in the small intestine or making them stronger, but without disrupting their rhythm.

Prophylactic: any medical or public health procedure whose purpose is to prevent, rather than treat or cure a disease. In general terms, prophylactic measures are divided between *primary* prophylaxis (to prevent the development of a disease) and *secondary* prophylaxis (whereby the disease has already developed and the patient is protected against worsening of this process).

Prostate: the prostate is a walnut-sized gland that forms part of the male reproductive system. The gland is made of two lobes, or regions, enclosed by an outer layer of tissue.

Prostatic hypertrophy: benign prostatic hyperplasia (BPH) also known as benign prostatic hypertrophy (technically a misnomer), benign enlargement of the prostate (BEP), and adenofibromyomatous hyperplasia, refers to the increase in size of the prostate.

Pulmonary embolism (PE): a blockage of the main artery of the lung or one of its branches by a substance that has travelled from elsewhere in the body.

Pulse oximeter: a medical device that indirectly monitors the oxygen saturation of a patient's blood (as opposed to measuring oxygen saturation directly).

Pupils (PEARRL): stands for Pupils Equal and Round, React to Light (used in assessing a patient's pupils).

Pyrazinamide: a drug used to treat tuberculosis. The drug is largely bacteriostatic, but can be bacteriocidal on actively replicating tuberculosis.

Ranitidine: a histamine H2-receptor antagonist that inhibits stomach acid production. It is commonly used in treatment of peptic ulcer disease (PUD).

Rapid response vehicles (RRV): emergency response vehicles can be used to reach a scene more quickly than a standard ambulance, as they may be able to move through traffic with greater ease, or travel at greater speed, to bring additional or more skilled resources to a scene, or simply to avoid sending too many resources to medical problems that do not require it.

Red flagged: a semi-official term to denote various attention and awareness indicators and signals, both explicit and implicit.

Rendezvous point (RVP): the designated meeting location away from the incident scene, where multi-agency resources are coordinated.

Resuscitation: an emergency procedure which is performed in an effort to manually preserve intact brain function until further measures are taken to restore spontaneous blood circulation and breathing in a person in cardiac arrest.

Rifampicin: an antibacterial and antifungal agent used in the treatment of mycobacterial infections.

RTC Road traffic collision: any incident involving pedestrian or vehicles on roads usually but not always a collision.

Salbutamol: a short-acting selective β_2-adrenoceptor stimulant delivered via an aerosol inhaler to control mild to moderate symptoms of asthma. Salbutamol relaxes the muscles which cause bronchial spasms in the lungs, the primary symptom of asthma.

Salmeterol: a β_2-adrenoceptor agonist used to control asthma and prevent pulmonary edema.

SAMPLE: for a focused history in emergency conditions and trauma this mnemonic is used:
S = signs and symptoms
A = allergies
M = medications
P = pertinent past medical history
L = last oral intake
E = events leading up to.
Helpful to remember key questions for a person's assessment.

Scooped: a colloquialism defining the handling of an orthopaedic scoop stretcher.

Secondary survey: this assessment is a complete examination of the patient from top to toe, both front and back. Divided into key areas: Head and Face, Neck, Chest, Abdomen, Back, Extremities and Neurological Examination.

Seizure: a sudden attack of illness, especially a stroke or an epileptic fit. An epileptic seizure, occasionally referred to as a fit, is defined as a transient symptom of 'abnormal excessive or synchronous neuronal activity in the brain'. The outward effect can be as dramatic as a wild thrashing movement (tonic-clonic seizure) or as mild as a brief loss of awareness.

Sepsis: the presence in tissues of harmful bacteria and their toxins, typically through infection of a wound. Sepsis is a serious medical condition that is characterized by a whole-body inflammatory state (called a systemic inflammatory response syndrome or SIRS) and the presence of a known or suspected infection.

Serum potassium: this test measures the amount of potassium in the blood. Potassium (K+) helps nerves and muscles communicate. Normal serum potassium levels are between 3.5 and 5.0 mEq/L; at least 95% of the body's potassium is found inside cells.

Sodium bicarbonate: a white crystalline weakly alkaline salt, $NaHCO_3$, used in baking powders and in medicine especially as an antacid – called also baking soda, bicarb, bicarbonate of soda, sodium acid carbonate.

Sodium chloride 0.9%: an aqueous solution of 0.9 per cent sodium chloride, isotonic with the blood and tissue fluid, used in medicine chiefly for bathing tissue and, in sterile form, as a solvent for drugs that are to be administered parenterally to replace body fluids. Use isotonic sodium chloride solution in a sentence.

Spider naevi: a painless skin condition formed by the dilation of a group of small blood vessels and characterized by a central and elevated red dot, about the size of a pinhead, from which small blood vessels radiate (looking like a spider).

Spironolactone: an aldosterone inhibitor that blocks the aldosterone-dependent exchange of sodium and potassium in the distal tubule, thus increasing excretion of sodium and water and decreasing excretion of potassium; used in the treatment of oedema, hypokalaemia, primary aldosteronism, and hypertension.

Splenomegaly: abnormal enlargement of the spleen.

Sputum: a mixture of saliva and mucus expectorated from the lungs and respiratory tract.

Standby: a holding position for ambulance crews between calls who have been instructed by control to wait for further instructions or emergency calls.

Status epilepticus: a condition in which there are continuing attacks of epilepsy without intervals of consciousness; can lead to brain damage and death.

STEMI: ST elevation myocardial infarction.

Stridor: a harsh vibrating noise when breathing, caused by obstruction of the windpipe or larynx.

Sulphonamides: any of a class of synthetic drugs, derived from sulfanilamide, that are able to prevent the multiplication of some pathogenic bacteria.

Temperature: the degree of internal heat of a person's body. The degree of hotness or coldness of a body or environment (corresponding to its molecular activity).

Tetracycline: any of a large group of antibiotics with a molecular structure containing four rings of carbon. A broad-spectrum polyketide antibiotic produced by the *Streptomyces* genus of Actinobacteria, indicated for use against many bacterial infections.

Thermoregulatory: thermoregulation is the ability of an organism to keep its body temperature within certain boundaries, even when the surrounding temperature is very different.

Thiamine (vitamin B1): a vitamin of the B complex, found in unrefined grains, beans, and liver, a deficiency of which causes beriberi. It is a sulphur-containing derivative of thiazole and pyrimidine.

Thrombophilia: thrombophilia or hypercoagulability is the propensity to develop thrombosis (blood clots) due to an abnormality in the system of coagulation.

Time critical: a seriously ill medical or trauma patient. A judgement call by the paramedic that they are required to get this patient to definitive care without undue delays.

Tonic-Clonic seizures: formerly known as grand mal seizures or gran mal seizures, these are a type of generalized seizure that affects the entire brain.

Transient ischaemic attack (TIA): this is caused by a temporary fall in the blood supply to part of the brain, leading to a lack of oxygen to the brain. This can cause symptoms that are similar to a stroke.

Triage: the process of determining the priority of patients' treatments based on the severity of their condition.

Tympanic temperature: the temperature readings are measured in the ear canal. The thermometers use infrared technology to measure body temperature.

Varices: dilated veins in the distal oesophagus or proximal stomach caused by elevated pressure in the portal venous system, typically from cirrhosis.

Vital signs: measures of various physiological statistics, often taken by health professionals, in order to assess the most basic body functions.

Volvulus: a bowel obstruction in which a loop of bowel has abnormally twisted on itself.

Warfarin: an anticoagulant used to prevent and treat the formation of harmful blood clots within the body by thinning the blood and/or dissolving clots.

Wernicke's encephalopathy: a syndrome characterized by ataxia, ophthalmoplegia, confusion, and impairment of short-term memory due to thiamine (vitamin B1) deficiency, also described as psychosis.

Wheezing: a high-pitched whistling sound during breathing. It occurs when air flows through narrowed breathing tubes, which is most obvious when breathing out (exhaling).

WHO (World Health Organization): WHO is the directing and coordinating authority for health within the United Nations system. It is responsible for providing leadership on global health matters, shaping the health research agenda, setting norms and standards, articulating evidence-based policy options, providing technical support to countries and monitoring and assessing health trends.

Index

Locators shown in *italics* refer to figures and tables.

159